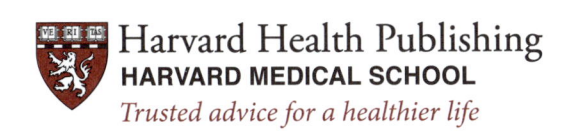

Dear Reader,

Welcome to the revised and updated edition of *Making Sense of Vitamins and Minerals: Choosing the foods and nutrients you need to stay healthy*. In the current version of the report, we provide the latest information to help you meet your vitamin and mineral needs—ideally through your diet rather than supplements. If you look at the list of vitamins and minerals you should consume every day, the goal of obtaining everything through your diet alone may seem daunting, but it's not as hard as it may sound. Globalization has created unprecedented access to an incredibly diverse food supply—including nutrient-rich fruits and vegetables—that past generations did not have. At the same time, however, a plethora of nutritionally poor foods and beverages (which also did not exist in times past) compete for your attention, bolstered through savvy labeling and purported health claims. As a result, it's more important than ever to be your own health advocate and to learn how to make wise nutritional choices.

Another feature of the current food landscape is the constant barrage of new studies that you read about in the media. Out of context, they may appear more conclusive than they really are. In updating this report, we help you make sense of the research on vitamins and minerals and provide you with the latest, most practical dietary strategies to ensure you get an adequate, but not excessive, intake of vitamins and minerals for your optimal health. We explain the many roles that vitamins and minerals play in your body, and give the recommended minimum and maximum amounts you should consume, as well as good food sources of each. We help you determine whether you are getting enough.

Where do supplements fit in? They remain as adjuncts to a healthy diet, not replacements for nutritious food. Although most U.S. adults take at least one vitamin and mineral supplement, the evidence remains inconclusive as to whether most of them confer health benefits. This report will help you decide whether or not to make them part of your dietary strategy. Among other things, you will learn

- what to look for when reading nutrition labels for foods and supplements
- why you might not be getting enough vitamin B_{12} from your diet
- how low levels of vitamin D might be detrimental to health
- the role of probiotics and prebiotics in keeping you healthy.

Yours in health,

Howard D. Sesso, Sc.D., M.P.H.
Medical Editor

Vitamins and minerals: The basics

Every day, your body produces new skin, muscle, and bone cells. It makes tens of thousands of rich red blood cells that carry nutrients and oxygen to every part of your body, and it produces multitudes of white blood cells to fight invaders. Your nerves send electrical signals skipping along thousands of miles of brain and body pathways, and your tissues formulate protein and fatty acid chemical messengers that shuttle from organ to organ, issuing the orders that orchestrate and sustain your life.

To do all this, your body requires many different raw materials. These include nearly 30 vitamins and minerals that your body cannot manufacture in sufficient amounts on its own. Acting in concert, these essential compounds perform thousands of roles in the body, ranging from shoring up bones and healing wounds to boosting your immune system, converting food into energy, and repairing cell and tissue damage.

The essential vitamins and minerals are often called micronutrients because your body needs only tiny amounts of them. (This is in contrast to the macronutrients—carbohydrates, fats, and protein—which the body requires in large amounts for energy, metabolism, and other functions.) Yet failing to get even those small quantities virtually guarantees disease. For example, British sailors learned centuries ago that living for months without fresh fruits or vegetables—the main sources of vitamin C—caused the bleeding gums and listlessness of scurvy, a disease that often proved fatal. Even today in many low-income countries, with limited access to healthy and diverse foods, people often suffer from a variety of nutrient-deficiency diseases, such as scurvy.

True vitamin and mineral deficiencies—in which the lack of a single nutrient leads directly to a specific ailment—are rare in the United States because of our extensive supply of inexpensive food and the fortification of many common foods with some key nutrients. However, eating less than optimal amounts of important vitamins, minerals, and other compounds can still contribute to a number of major illnesses, such as heart disease, type 2 diabetes, cancer, and osteoporosis. Hence, concern about "nutritional insufficiency"— a controversial topic—is a major driver of both the U.S. dietary guidelines and the mass marketing of over-the-counter supplements.

So how can you make sure you're fulfilling your nutrient needs? Unfortunately, a welter of conflicting studies has led to general confusion—and all too many studies lead to new marketing claims that may or may not be upheld by later research. In fact, the best way to get vitamins and minerals is from a well-rounded diet, with plenty of fruits, vegetables, legumes, whole grains, and lean sources of protein, along with healthy fats, such as nuts and olive oil.

We'll explore all of this in this report. But first, it may help

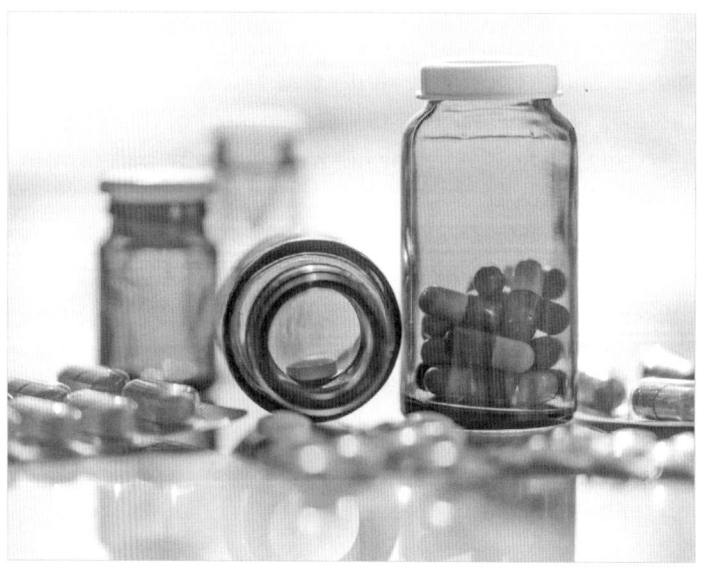

It is rare in this country to encounter true vitamin deficiencies, such as the disease scurvy, which is caused by lack of vitamin C. But many people get less than optimal levels of key micronutrients.

to review some important differences between vitamins and minerals and their roles in the body.

Vitamins vs. minerals

What distinguishes a vitamin from a mineral? A vitamin, simply put, is an organic substance—one produced by a plant or an animal—that is required in small amounts for human life. (The first syllable, *vit-*, comes from the Latin word for "life.") With the exception of vitamin D, vitamins cannot be synthesized in the body and must come from food. They are therefore considered essential micronutrients.

A mineral is an inorganic element—one that comes originally from rocks, soil, or water (though it may enter your diet through a plant that has absorbed it from the environment, or an animal that has eaten such a plant). There are many minerals, but only certain ones are necessary for human health.

Another difference is that vitamins have complex structures that can be broken down by heat, air, or acid. Minerals are simpler elements that hold on to their chemical structures. That means minerals can easily find their way into your body through the plants, fish, animals, and fluids you consume. It's more difficult to shuttle vitamins from food into your body, because cooking, storage, and simple exposure to air can inactivate these more fragile compounds.

Despite their differences, vitamins and minerals often work together. For example, vitamin D enables your body to pluck calcium from food that is passing through your digestive tract, rather than harvesting it from your own bones. Vitamin C helps you absorb iron. However, the interplay of micronutrients isn't always cooperative. For example, too much vitamin C can block your body's ability to assimilate the essential mineral copper.

There are a couple other distinctions to be aware of. Vitamins are subdivided into two categories—water-soluble and fat-soluble—with implications for your diet. Minerals, too, are subdivided into major minerals and trace minerals, depending on how much you need of each. Many vitamins and some minerals are also classified as antioxidants. This chapter will explore these concepts in greater depth.

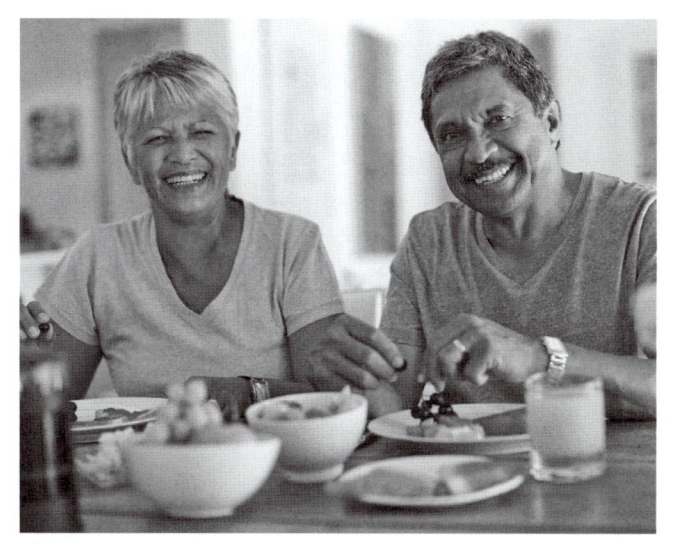

The best way to get vitamins and minerals is from a well-rounded diet, with plenty of fruits, vegetables, and whole grains.

Water-soluble vitamins

Water-soluble vitamins—those that can dissolve in water—are packed into the watery portions of the foods you eat. They are absorbed directly from the digestive tract into the bloodstream as food is broken down or as a supplement dissolves. (For this reason, you should consume water-soluble vitamin supplements with food to ensure full absorption.) Because much of your body consists of water, many of the water-soluble vitamins circulate easily in your body. One exception is vitamin B_6, which is mostly stored in muscle tissue.

Your kidneys continuously regulate levels of water-soluble vitamins, shunting excesses out of the body in your urine. Because of this, the risk of harm from consuming supplements that contain large doses of these vitamins is relatively small in most cases. However, there are some exceptions. For example, excessive vitamin B_6 (many times the recommended daily amount

▶ **Water-soluble vitamins**

B vitamins:
- Biotin (vitamin B_7)
- Folic acid (folate, vitamin B_9)
- Niacin (vitamin B_3)
- Pantothenic acid (vitamin B_5)
- Riboflavin (vitamin B_2)
- Thiamin (vitamin B_1)
- Vitamin B_6
- Vitamin B_{12}

Vitamin C

of 1.3 milligrams for adults) can damage nerves, causing numbness and muscle weakness (see "B bonanza: Boon or bust?" on page 21).

Although water-soluble vitamins tend to pass out of the body quickly, some can stay for long periods of time. You probably have several years' supply of vitamin B12 in your liver. Even folic acid and vitamin C stores can last more than a couple of days. Generally, though, water-soluble vitamins should be replenished every few days.

Water-soluble vitamins perform many tasks in the body. One of the most important is helping to free the energy found in the food you eat. Thiamin, riboflavin, niacin, pantothenic acid, and biotin—all of them B vitamins—engage in various aspects of energy production. Vitamins B6, B12, and folic acid metabolize amino acids (the building blocks of proteins) and help cells multiply. And one of many roles played by vitamin C is to help make collagen, which knits together wounds, supports blood vessel walls, and forms a base for teeth and bones.

Figure 1: Absorption of fat-soluble vitamins

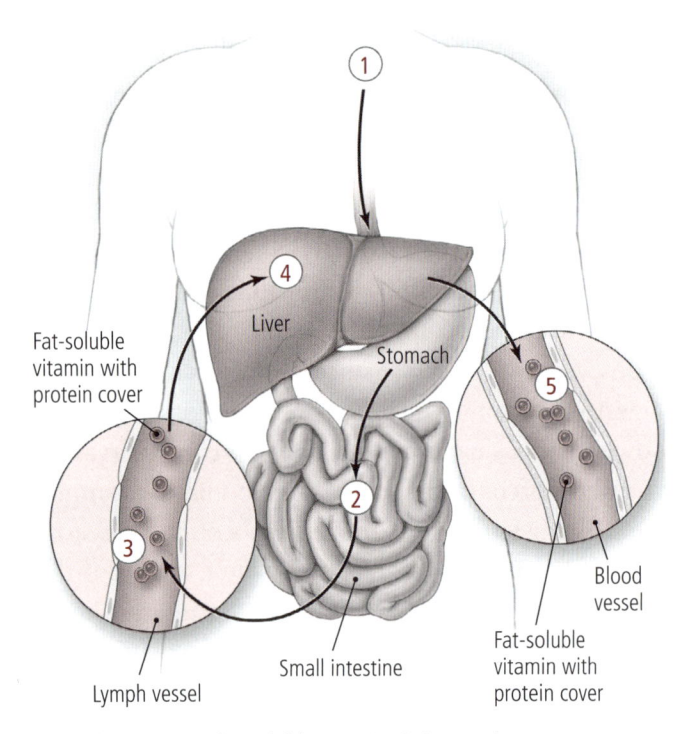

1. Food containing fat-soluble vitamins is ingested.

2. The food is broken down by stomach acid and then travels to the small intestine, where it is digested further. Bile is needed for the absorption of fat-soluble vitamins. This substance, which is produced in the liver, flows into the small intestine, where it breaks down fats. Nutrients are then absorbed through the wall of the small intestine.

3. Upon absorption, the fat-soluble vitamins enter the lymph vessels before making their way into the bloodstream. In most cases, fat-soluble vitamins must be coupled with a protein—which is why they should be taken with food and not alone—in order to travel through the body.

4. These vitamins are used throughout the body, but excesses are stored in the liver and fat tissues.

5. As additional amounts of these vitamins are needed, your body taps into the reserves, and the liver releases them into the bloodstream.

Fat-soluble vitamins

As the name implies, fat-soluble vitamins can be dissolved by fat solvents and oils. In contrast to water-soluble vitamins, which easily move from the bloodstream into your cells and are excreted in urine, fat-soluble vitamins need special ways to move around the body. After being consumed in the diet, fat-soluble vitamins gain entry to the bloodstream via lymph channels in the intestinal wall (see Figure 1, at left). Most fat-soluble vitamins travel through the body only under the escort of special fat-binding proteins, which act as carriers to allow these vitamins to interact with water-rich blood and cells.

Together the fat-soluble vitamins keep many parts of your body in good repair. For example, vitamins A, D, and K are essential for bone formation. Vitamin A also helps keep cells healthy and protects your vision—but without vitamin E, the fourth fat-soluble vitamin, your body would have difficulty absorbing and storing vitamin A. Vitamin E also acts as an antioxidant, potentially helping to protect your cells and even your DNA against damage from unstable molecules called free radicals (see "Understanding antioxidants," page 6).

Fat-soluble vitamins are stored in your fat tissues and your liver, which together

▶ **Fat-soluble vitamins**
- Vitamin A
- Vitamin D
- Vitamin E
- Vitamin K

4   Making Sense of Vitamins and Minerals   www.health.harvard.edu

act as the main holding pens for these vitamins and release them as needed. To some extent, you can think of these vitamins as time-release nutrients. Your body squirrels away any excess you consume and doles it out gradually to meet your needs. Because these vitamins are stored for long periods, however, dangerous levels can build up. As a result, potential toxicity from fat-soluble vitamins is much more common than for water-soluble vitamins. However, this is most likely to happen if you take high doses of supplements over a prolonged period of time. It's very rare to get too much of any vitamin just from food.

Major minerals

The body needs and stores relatively large amounts of the major minerals—calcium, chloride, magnesium, potassium, phosphorus, sodium, and sulfur. Calcium and phosphorus each account for more than a pound of your body weight. One of the key tasks of the major minerals is maintaining the proper electrical balance of all the cell membranes in your body—an essential property for cell signaling and the transport of nutrients and messengers into and out of cells. Sodium, chloride, and potassium take the lead in doing this. Three other major minerals—calcium, phosphorus, and magnesium—have similar activities and are also important for healthy bones. Sulfur helps stabilize protein structures, including some of those that make up hair, skin, and nails.

Major minerals travel through the body in various ways. Potassium, for example, is quickly absorbed into the bloodstream, where it circulates freely and is excreted by the kidneys, much like a water-soluble vitamin. In contrast, calcium requires a carrier for absorption and transport.

Having too much of one major mineral can result in a deficiency of another. Calcium binds with excess sodium in the body and is excreted when the body senses that sodium levels must be lowered. That means that if you ingest too much sodium through table salt or processed foods, you could end up losing needed calcium as your body rids itself of the surplus sodium. Likewise, too much phosphorus can hamper your ability to absorb magnesium. These sorts of imbalances are usually caused by overloads from supplements, not food sources.

Trace minerals

A thimble could easily contain all the trace minerals normally found in your body. Yet their contributions are just as essential as those of the major minerals. Trace minerals carry out a diverse set of tasks. Iron, for example, is best known for ferrying oxygen throughout the body, while fluoride strengthens bones and wards off tooth decay. Zinc helps your blood clot, is essential for taste and smell, and bolsters your immune response. Copper helps form several enzymes, one of which assists with iron metabolism and the creation of hemoglobin, which carries oxygen in the blood. The other trace minerals perform equally vital jobs, such as helping to block damage to body cells and forming parts of key enzymes or enhancing their activity.

Trace minerals interact with one another, sometimes in ways that can trigger imbalances. Too much of one can cause or contribute to a deficiency of another. For example, a minor overload of manganese can worsen an iron deficiency. By the same token, too little of a mineral can lead to health problems. When the body has too little iodine, thyroid hormone production slows, causing sluggishness and weight gain as well as other health concerns. The problem worsens if the body also has too little selenium.

However, the difference between "just enough" and "too much" of the trace minerals is often relatively small. Generally, food is a safe source of trace minerals, but if you take supple-

> **Major minerals**
> - Calcium
> - Chloride
> - Magnesium
> - Phosphorus
> - Potassium
> - Sodium
> - Sulfur

> **Trace minerals**
> - Chromium
> - Copper
> - Fluoride
> - Iodine
> - Iron
> - Manganese
> - Molybdenum
> - Selenium
> - Zinc

ments, it's important to make sure you're not greatly exceeding recommended levels.

Understanding antioxidants

Some vitamins and minerals—including vitamins C and E and the minerals copper, zinc, and selenium—serve as antioxidants, in addition to other vital roles.

"Antioxidant" is a general term for any compound that can counteract unstable molecules called free radicals that damage DNA, cell membranes, and other parts of cells. Because free radicals lack a full complement of electrons, they steal electrons from other molecules and damage those molecules in the process. Antioxidants neutralize free radicals by giving up some of their own electrons. In making this sacrifice, they act as a natural "off" switch for the free radicals. This helps break a chain reaction that can affect other molecules in the cell and other cells in the body. But it is important to recognize that the term "antioxidant" reflects a chemical property rather than a specific nutritional property.

While free radicals are damaging by their very nature, they are an inescapable part of life. The body generates free radicals in response to environmental insults, such as tobacco smoke, ultraviolet rays, and air pollution, but they are also a natural byproduct of normal processes in cells. When the immune system musters to fight intruders, for example, the oxygen it uses spins off an army of free radicals that destroy viruses, bacteria, and damaged body cells in an oxidative burst. Some normal production of free radicals also occurs during exercise. This appears to be necessary in order to induce some of the beneficial effects of regular physical activity, such as sensitizing your muscle cells to insulin.

Because free radicals are so pervasive, you need an adequate supply of antioxidants to disarm them. Your body's cells naturally produce some powerful antioxidants, such as alpha lipoic acid and glutathione. The foods you eat supply other antioxidants, such as vitamins C and E. Plants are full of compounds known as phytochemicals—literally, "plant chemicals"—many of which seem to have antioxidant properties as well. For example, after vitamin C has "quenched" a free radical by donating electrons to it, a phytochemical called hesperetin (found in oranges and other citrus fruits) restores the vitamin C to its active antioxidant form. Carotenoids (such as lycopene in tomatoes and lutein in kale) and flavonoids (such as flavanols in cocoa, anthocyanins in blueberries, quercetin in apples and onions, and catechins in green tea) are also antioxidants.

News articles, advertisements, and food labels often tout antioxidants as a way to help slow aging, fend off heart disease, improve flagging vision, and curb cancer. And laboratory studies and many large-scale observational studies (those that query people about their eating habits and supplement use and then track their disease patterns) have noted benefits from diets rich in antioxidants, particularly those coming from a broad range of colorful vegetables and fruits. But results from randomized controlled trials of antioxidant supplements (in which people are assigned to take specific nutrient supplements or a placebo) have not supported many of these claims. (See "Making sense of scientific studies," page 15, for more detail on the types of research studies and why their results often differ.) Indeed, too much of these antioxidant supplements won't help you and may even harm you. It is better to supply your antioxidants from a well-rounded diet.

Understanding the federal guidelines

The field of nutrition is filled with confusing terms—Recommended Dietary Allowances (RDAs), Daily Values (DVs), dietary reference intakes (DRIs), and more. However, few people aside from nutritionists really understand the differences between these terms. To help you sort through it all, this chapter traces the history of the terms and explains why the different values are used in different situations.

Recommended Dietary Allowances

In 1941, the U.S. Food and Nutrition Board published the first in a series of reports on Recommended Dietary Allowances (RDAs). These reports were directly inspired by concern about nutrient deficiencies, which in the early 20th century were still relatively common in the United States, and which the government and nutrition experts worried could be worsened by food shortages caused by the Great Depression and World War II. The RDAs in turn were used as the foundation for the first U.S. Dietary Guidelines for Americans. These guidelines are revised every five years to reflect advances in nutrition knowledge. (The latest version was released in late 2015, and the next iteration is due in 2020.)

This process—setting RDAs based on concern about potential nutrient deficiencies, and then basing the dietary guidelines on these standards—has continued with relatively little change since the 1940s. Although this has contributed to success at largely eliminating nutrient deficiencies in the United States, it has also had unintended consequences. The isolated focus of the RDAs on single nutrients—which works so well for preventing diseases like rickets or scurvy that are caused by a lack of single nutrients—has questionable relevance for staving off heart disease, cancer, and other chronic diseases.

Figure 2: A sample Nutrition Facts panel

Nearly every packaged food or beverage you toss into your shopping cart has a printed Nutrition Facts panel, which includes a mandated list of selected nutrients contained in the product. This includes the gram or milligram amounts and the percentages of Daily Values (reference numbers designed to help consumers determine if a food contains a lot or a little of a specific nutrient) in a single serving of the food or drink. It also includes other information such as serving size, calories per serving, and amounts of fat, cholesterol, sodium, carbohydrate, and protein. Beyond that, there is some limited information about vitamins and minerals.

In 2016, the FDA updated the label to keep up with advances in nutrition science and to make the nutrition information easier for consumers to understand. Large manufacturers (those with $10 million or more in annual sales) are required to be printing the new label on all products by Jan. 1, 2020; smaller manufacturers (those selling less than $10 million annually) have until Jan. 1, 2021, to change their labels.

The new label is very similar to the old label, but it lists calories and serving size in a larger type size. Manufacturers must also state how much sugar—both total sugar and added sugars (those that are added during processing)—are in a product, along with how much calcium, iron, vitamin D, and potassium it contains. Vitamins A and C, which used to be required, needn't be listed, but can be included if the manufacturer would like to list them. Producers can also include information on other vitamins and minerals at their discretion.

Nutrition Facts
8 servings per container
Serving size 2/3 cup (55g)

Amount per serving
Calories 230

	% Daily Value*
Total Fat 8g	10%
Saturated Fat 1g	5%
Trans Fat 0g	
Cholesterol 0mg	0%
Sodium 160mg	7%
Total Carbohydrate 37g	13%
Dietary Fiber 4g	14%
Total Sugars 12g	
Includes 10g Added Sugars	20%
Protein 3g	
Vitamin D 2mcg	10%
Calcium 260mg	20%
Iron 8mg	45%
Potassium 235mg	6%

* The % Daily Value (DV) tells you how much a nutrient in a serving of food contributes to a daily diet. 2,000 calories a day is used for general nutrition advice.

The establishment of RDAs is now a highly complex—and expensive—process. New RDAs, or even a revised value for an existing RDA, can be determined by only one private, nonprofit agency—known as the Health and Medicine Division of the National Academies of Sciences, Engineering, and Medicine—and only after it receives a special commission and special funding from the U.S. government. The process is lengthy and pricey, taking up to three years and millions of dollars to revise a single RDA. As a result, such revisions are infrequent. The most recent RDA revision—for vitamin D and calcium—was published in 2011, when the Health and Medicine Division was known as the Institute of Medicine, or IOM (see "How much vitamin D do you need?" on page 24).

Because RDAs were designed to prevent clinical nutrient deficiencies, they apply only to a limited set of nutrients and their corresponding nutrient deficiency diseases. To create guidelines for appropriate intakes of other nutrients, other criteria have been developed, such as adequate intakes, or AIs (see "Alphabet soup: Making sense of RDAs, DRIs, DVs, and other values," below). Together, these sets of criteria for nutrient consumption are called dietary reference intakes (DRIs). The DRIs are intended to be evidence-based standards that go beyond amending single-nutrient deficiencies: they also suggest the amounts of nutrients needed for preventing complex chronic diseases and enhancing health.

To help people apply these vitamin and mineral guidelines to their daily food choices, the FDA created the Nutrition Facts panel that appears on almost all packaged foods (see Figure 2, page 7). This panel was recently updated.

When you read nutrition labels, bear in mind that the limited information on vitamin and mineral content is only one factor to consider. Other factors—for example, the extent of food processing, the quality of the carbohydrates, and the types of fat—are just as important, if not more important. To glean all this from

Alphabet soup: Making sense of RDAs, DRIs, DVs, and other values

Recommended Dietary Allowances (RDAs) are the nutrition labeling guidelines established in the 1940s. But how do they differ from DRIs and DVs? And what are ULs and AIs? Here's some help.

Recommended Dietary Allowance (RDA): This value refers to the average minimum amount of a specific nutrient needed to prevent clinical nutrient deficiency in almost all healthy people in a particular life stage and gender group. Because RDAs apply to only a selected set of nutrients and nutrient deficiency diseases, today RDAs are a subset of the broader dietary reference intake values (see below).

Dietary reference intake (DRI): Introduced in 1997, DRI values were created to support guidelines for a broader range of nutrients and minerals, not only to prevent nutrient deficiencies, but also to enhance health and reduce the risk of chronic diseases such as osteoporosis, cancer, and cardiovascular disease. DRIs include RDAs, AIs, ULs, and EARs (see the next three entries). DRIs are what underlie the U.S. dietary guidelines and food labeling regulations.

Adequate intake (AI): This value is determined as a range of recommended intake (rather than just a minimum), and is used for nutrients for which there is not a specific clinical deficiency disease, such as vitamin K, manganese, and potassium.

Tolerable upper intake level (UL): This is the maximum amount of a nutrient that is considered safe for individuals—including those in sensitive subgroups—to consume daily for an extended period. Exceeding the UL does not mean that harmful effects will always occur; rather, the more a person exceeds the UL, the greater the risk of adverse effects.

Estimated average requirement (EAR): This is the amount of a nutrient that is estimated to meet the requirement of half of all healthy people in a particular life stage and gender group to prevent clinical nutrient deficiency. EARs are used as the basis for RDAs, and as such, apply to a relatively limited set of nutrients and their corresponding nutrient deficiency diseases.

Daily Value (DV): This reference number, developed by the FDA, is designed to help consumers determine if a food contains a lot or a little of a specific nutrient, based on the DRI for that nutrient. It may be similar to the RDA or AI for that nutrient, but not always. DVs—which are used on Nutrition Facts panels—don't take into account your age, sex, or other factors affecting your daily calorie needs. They're based on the highest average daily allowance value and are presented as percentages of total daily intake, calculated for an average person eating 2,000 calories a day.

Note: Another point of confusion can be the units used for measuring various vitamins and minerals. Amounts may be presented as milligrams (mg), micrograms (mcg), or international units (IU). To convert one to the other, consult this calculator: www.health.harvard.edu/iu-converter.

the Nutrition Facts panel requires a little interpretation. For example, to assess carbohydrate quality, a rule of thumb is to look for no more than 10 grams of total carbohydrate for every 1 gram of fiber (a 10-to-1 ratio or lower). In the label shown in Figure 2 (page 7), there are 37 grams of carbohydrate and 4 grams of fiber, making the ratio 37 to 4, or slightly less than 10 to 1. Looking for a 10-to-1 ratio is not a perfect rule of thumb, but it helps to capture the overall quality of the carbohydrate in any product. If you really want to maximize carbohydrate quality, aim for a 5-to-1 ratio—in other words, no more than 5 grams of carbohydrate for every 1 gram of fiber.

But even more important than the carbohydrate quality or fat content of one particular food is your overall dietary pattern. If you eat a diverse assortment of whole, minimally processed foods—fruits, vegetables, nuts, whole grains, fish, vegetable oils, and modest amounts of dairy—there's little need to become a nutrition label mathematician. You're already getting high-quality macronutrients (fats, carbs, and protein), as well as plenty of vitamins and minerals.

Tables 1 and 2, starting below, can give you a better understanding of how particular vitamins and minerals work in your body, how much of each nutrient you need every day, and what types of food to eat to ensure that you are getting an adequate supply. When reading the tables, note the following:

- The recommendations vary by age and sex. These

Table 1: Vitamins: Recommended intake, uses in the body, and sources

The following recommendations are based largely on guidelines from the Health and Medicine Division of the National Academies. Recommended amounts may be expressed in milligrams (mg), micrograms (mcg), or international units (IU), depending on the nutrient. Unless specified, values represent those for men (M) and women (W) ages 19 and older.

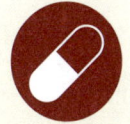

VITAMIN AND BENEFITS	RDA OR AI*	UL*	GOOD FOOD SOURCES (listed most to least)	DID YOU KNOW?
Vitamin A (retinol, retinal, and retinoic acid—three active forms of vitamin A in the body—are retinoids, called "preformed" vitamin A; the body can also easily convert a precursor, beta carotene, to vitamin A as needed) • Essential for vision • Keeps tissues and skin healthy • Plays an important role in bone growth	RDA M: 3,000 IU (900 mcg) W: 2,333 IU (700 mcg)	10,000 IU (3,000 mcg)	*Sources of preformed vitamin A:* beef liver, ricotta cheese, Atlantic herring, fortified milk and cereal *Sources of beta carotene:* sweet potatoes, spinach, carrots, pumpkin, cantaloupe, peppers, mangoes	Large amounts of supplemental, or preformed, vitamin A (but not beta carotene) can be harmful to bones. In current smokers, beta carotene supplements may raise the risk of lung cancer.
Thiamin (thiamine, vitamin B1) • Helps convert food into energy • Needed for healthy skin, hair, muscles, and brain	RDA M: 1.2 mg W: 1.1 mg	Not known	Fortified cereals, pork chops, rice, trout, black beans, mussels, tuna, acorn squash	Thiamin deficiency can occur with chronic, heavy alcohol consumption, leading to a condition called Wernicke-Korsakoff syndrome.
Riboflavin (vitamin B2) • Helps convert food into energy • Needed for healthy skin, hair, blood, and brain	RDA M: 1.3 mg W: 1.1 mg	Not known	Beef liver, fortified cereals and oats, yogurt, milk, beef, clams, almonds, cheese	Most Americans get the RDA for riboflavin, mostly from milk and milk-based beverages. Riboflavin is destroyed by light, which is why most milk is sold in opaque containers.
Niacin (vitamin B3, nicotinic acid) • Helps convert food into energy • Essential for healthy skin, blood cells, brain, and nervous system	RDA M: 16 mg W: 14 mg	35 mg	Fortified cereals, baker's yeast, salmon, tuna, beef, lamb, peanuts and peanut butter, chicken, veal, mushrooms, turkey	Niacin occurs naturally in food and can also be made by your body from the amino acid tryptophan, with the help of B6.
Pantothenic acid (vitamin B5) • Helps convert food into energy • Helps make lipids (fats), neurotransmitters, steroid hormones, and hemoglobin	AI 5 mg	Not known	Wide variety of foods, including fortified cereals, beef liver, mushrooms, sunflower seeds, chicken, tuna, avocados	The name pantothenic comes from the Greek word *pantothen*, meaning "from all sides"—a nod to its wide availability in many foods. Deficiencies are very rare.

continued

tables apply to adults ages 19 and over. If you are looking for recommendations for someone younger, or for a pregnant or nursing woman, ask your doctor about what's appropriate.

- The recommended amount for each nutrient is either an RDA (if there is a deficiency disease, such as rickets or pellagra, associated with it) or an AI (for most other nutrients; see "Alphabet soup: Making sense of RDAs, DRIs, DVs, and other values," page 8).

Table 1 *continued*

VITAMIN AND BENEFITS	RDA OR AI*	UL*	GOOD FOOD SOURCES (listed most to least)	DID YOU KNOW?
Vitamin B6 (pyridoxal, pyridoxine, pyridoxamine) • Aids in lowering homocysteine levels; not clear whether it reduces heart disease risk • Helps convert tryptophan to niacin and serotonin, a neurotransmitter that plays key roles in sleep, appetite, and moods • Helps make red blood cells • Influences cognitive abilities and immune function	RDA Ages 19 to 50: 1.3 mg M, ages 51+: 1.7 mg W, ages 51+: 1.5 mg	100 mg	Chickpeas, beef liver, tuna, salmon, chicken breast, fortified cereals, potatoes, turkey, banana, marinara sauce, ground beef, waffles, bulgur, cottage cheese, winter squash	Vitamin B6 has been promoted as a treatment for carpal tunnel syndrome and premenstrual syndrome, but studies do not support any benefit for these conditions.
Biotin (vitamin B7) • Helps convert food into energy and synthesize glucose • Helps make and break down some fatty acids • Needed for healthy bones and hair	AI 30 mcg	Not known	Organ meats such as beef liver and eggs are good sources; also found in lesser concentration in fish, pork, hamburgers, sunflower seeds, sweet potatoes, and almonds	Your body needs very little biotin. Some is made by bacteria in the gastrointestinal tract. However, it's not clear how much of this the body absorbs.
Folic acid (vitamin B9, folate, folacin) • Vital for new cell creation • Helps prevent brain and spinal birth defects when taken early in pregnancy • Can lower levels of homocysteine; not clear whether it reduces heart disease risk • May reduce risk for colon cancer • Offsets breast cancer risk among women who consume alcohol	RDA 400 mcg	1,000 mcg	Beef liver, spinach, black-eyed peas, fortified grains and cereals, rice, asparagus, spaghetti, romaine lettuce, avocado, broccoli, mustard greens, green peas, kidney beans, peanuts, wheat germ	It's easier to absorb folic acid from supplements and fortified grain products than from foods where it occurs naturally. It should be taken regularly by all women of childbearing age, since deficiencies very early in pregnancy can lead to birth defects, and women may not know they are pregnant in the first weeks of pregnancy. Some research suggests that these women should get 800 mcg per day. You can get this amount through a healthy diet and a daily multivitamin. Rarely, folic acid masks a B12 deficiency, which can lead to severe neurological complications. That's not a reason to avoid folic acid; just be sure to get enough B12.
Vitamin B12 (cyanocobalamin) • Aids in lowering homocysteine levels; not clear whether it lowers heart disease risk • Assists in making new cells and breaking down some fatty acids and amino acids • Protects nerve cells and encourages their normal growth • Helps make red blood cells	RDA 2.4 mcg	Not known	Clams, beef liver, fortified cereals, fish (such as trout, salmon, tuna, and haddock), beef sirloin, milk, yogurt, cheese, ham, eggs	Many people, particularly older adults, are deficient in vitamin B12 because they have trouble absorbing this vitamin from food. Vitamin B12 occurs naturally only in animal food sources, so strict vegetarians and vegans should take a multivitamin to get enough. A lack of vitamin B12 can cause memory loss, dementia, and numbness in the arms and legs.

continued

- Pay attention to the column that lists the UL, which is the tolerable upper intake level. This is the maximum daily amount of a nutrient considered safe if consumed regularly. Beyond that limit, there is a rising risk for side effects, some of which can be serious. An upper limit hasn't been established for some nutrients; however, it's important to realize that very large amounts of these nutrients could still be harmful. Food sources of nutrients are almost never a problem. People run into trouble mostly through taking high doses of supplements.
- A good food source, as determined by the FDA, indicates a food that contains 10% to 19% of the RDA or AI of a specific nutrient.

Table 1 *continued*

VITAMIN AND BENEFITS	RDA OR AI*	UL*	GOOD FOOD SOURCES (listed most to least)	DID YOU KNOW?
Vitamin C (ascorbic acid) • Helps make collagen, a connective tissue that knits together wounds and supports blood vessel walls • Helps make the neurotransmitters serotonin and norepinephrine • Acts as an antioxidant, neutralizing unstable molecules that can damage cells • Bolsters the immune system	RDA M: 90 mg W: 75 mg Smokers: add 35 mg	3,000 mg	Red peppers, oranges and orange juice, grapefruit and grapefruit juice, kiwifruit, green peppers, broccoli, strawberries, Brussels sprouts, tomato juice, cantaloupe, cabbage, cauliflower, potatoes, tomatoes, spinach, green peas	Megadoses of vitamin C do not appear to help prevent the common cold, and they may cause diarrhea. Large-scale randomized clinical trials of vitamin C have not found an effect on cardiovascular disease and cancer.
Vitamin D (calciferol) • Helps ensure dietary calcium is absorbed into the body • Helps maintain normal blood levels of calcium and phosphorus, which strengthen bones • Helps form teeth and bones • Contributes to immune function • Supplements can reduce the number of nonvertebral fractures	RDA Ages 1 to 70: 600 IU (15 mcg) Ages 71+: 800 IU (20 mcg)	4,000 IU (100 mcg)	Cod liver oil, swordfish, salmon, tuna, fortified milk, cereals, and juices, sardines, beef liver, eggs	Some Americans, especially African Americans, don't get enough of this nutrient. The major source is sunlight, not diet. (Your skin naturally makes vitamin D when exposed to the sun.) While the body uses sunlight to make vitamin D, it may not make enough if you live in northern climates. Vitamin D has been suggested to have a wide range of benefits on health outcomes, yet randomized clinical trials have not yet produced definitive results. Trials are in progress.
Vitamin E (alpha tocopherol) • Acts as an antioxidant, neutralizing unstable molecules that can damage cells • Protects vitamin A and certain lipids from damage	RDA 22 IU (15 mg)	1,500 IU (1,000 mg)	Wheat germ oil, sunflower seeds and oil, almonds, safflower oil, hazelnuts, peanut butter and peanuts, corn oil, spinach	Vitamin E does not prevent wrinkles; the extent of its benefits, if any, is unclear. Vitamin E has been suggested to have numerous health benefits, but based on clinical trials, experts recommend against consuming supplements to prevent cancer or cardiovascular disease.
Vitamin K (phylloquinone, menadione) • Activates proteins and calcium essential to blood clotting • May help prevent hip fractures	AI M: 120 mcg W: 90 mcg	Not known	Collards, turnip greens, spinach, kale broccoli, soybeans and soybean oil, carrot juice, edamame, pumpkin, pomegranate juice, okra, salad dressing, pine nuts, blueberries, iceberg lettuce, chicken breast, grapes, vegetable juice cocktail, canola oil, cashews, carrots, olive oil	Intestinal bacteria make a form of vitamin K that accounts for half of your requirements. If you take an anticoagulant, keep your vitamin K intake consistent.

*RDA = Recommended Dietary Allowance; AI = adequate intake; UL = tolerable upper intake level.

Table 2: Minerals: Recommended intake, uses in the body, and sources

MINERAL AND BENEFITS	RDA OR AI*	UL*	GOOD FOOD SOURCES (listed most to least)	DID YOU KNOW?
Calcium • Builds and protects bones and teeth • Helps with muscle contractions and relaxation, blood clotting, and nerve impulse transmission • Plays a role in hormone secretion and enzyme activation • Helps maintain healthy blood pressure	RDA Men, ages 19 to 70: 1,000 mg Men, ages 71+: 1,200 mg Women, ages 19 to 50: 1,000 mg Women, ages 51+: 1,200 mg	Ages 19 to 50: 2,500 mg Ages 51+: 2,000 mg	Yogurt, cheese, sardines, milk, soymilk, fortified juices, tofu, salmon, frozen yogurt, and leafy green vegetables such as turnip greens, kale, and broccoli (but not spinach or Swiss chard, which have binders that lessen absorption)	Adults absorb roughly 30% of calcium ingested, but this can vary depending on the source. Some physicians recommend that pregnant women get more calcium than the current RDA. Ask your own doctor for advice.
Chloride • Balances fluids in the body • A component of stomach acid, essential to digestion	AI Ages 19 to 50: 2,300 mg Ages 51 to 70: 2,000 mg Ages 71+: 1,800 mg	3,600 mg	Salt (sodium chloride), soy sauce, processed foods, seaweed, rye, tomatoes, lettuce, celery, and olives	Chloride, sodium, and potassium help your body maintain the proper balance of water.
Chromium • Enhances the activity of insulin • Helps maintain normal blood glucose levels • Helps free energy from glucose	AI M, ages 19 to 50: 35 mcg M, ages 51+: 30 mcg W, ages 19 to 50: 25 mcg W, ages 51+: 20 mcg	Not known	Broccoli, potatoes, apples, orange juice, whole grain bread, beef, garlic, basil	Most foods provide just small amounts of chromium (less than 2 mcg per serving). Meats, whole-grain foods, and some fruits, vegetables, and spices are the best sources of chromium.
Copper • Plays an important role in iron metabolism • Helps make red blood cells	RDA 900 mcg	10,000 mcg	Liver, shellfish, nuts, seeds, whole-grain products, beans, prunes, cocoa	The body absorbs more than half of dietary copper in the gastrointestinal tract, and deficiency is not known to occur in adults.
Fluoride • Encourages strong bone formation • Keeps dental cavities from starting or worsening	AI M: 4 mg W: 3 mg	10 mg	Water that is fluoridated, toothpaste with fluoride, teas	Excessive amounts of fluoride are harmful to children.
Iodine • Part of thyroid hormone, which helps set body temperature and influences nerve and muscle function, reproduction, and growth • Prevents goiter and a congenital thyroid disorder in children	RDA 150 mcg	1,100 mcg	Seaweed, fish, yogurt, iodized salt, enriched bread, shrimp, ice cream, pasta, eggs, tuna	To prevent iodine deficiencies, some countries add iodine to salt, bread, or drinking water.

continued

Table 2 *continued*

MINERAL AND BENEFITS	RDA OR AI*	UL*	GOOD FOOD SOURCES (listed most to least)	DID YOU KNOW?
Iron • Helps hemoglobin in red blood cells and myoglobin in muscle cells ferry oxygen throughout the body • Needed for chemical reactions in the body and for making amino acids, collagen, neurotransmitters, and hormones	RDA M, ages 19 to 50: 8 mg M, ages 51+: 8 mg W, ages 19 to 50: 18 mg W, ages 51+: 8 mg	45 mg	Fortified breakfast cereals, oysters, beans, dark chocolate, beef liver, lentils, spinach, tofu, sardines, chickpeas, tomatoes, beef, potatoes, nuts	Many women of childbearing age don't get enough iron. Eating meat, fish, or poultry with beans or dark leafy greens can boost your absorption of vegetable sources of iron up to three times. Foods rich in vitamin C can also increase iron absorption.
Magnesium • Needed for many chemical reactions in the body • Works with calcium in muscle contraction, blood clotting, and regulation of blood pressure; may help protect against heart disease • Helps build bones and teeth	RDA M, ages 19 to 30: 400 mg M, ages 31+: 420 mg W, ages 19 to 30: 310 mg W, ages 31+: 320 mg	350 mg (Note: This upper limit applies to supplements and medicines, such as laxatives, not to dietary magnesium.)	Nuts, spinach, cereal, soymilk, black beans, edamame, peanut butter, bread, avocados, potatoes, rice, yogurt, fortified breakfast cereals	Many Americans don't get the required amounts. The majority of magnesium in the body is found in bones. If your blood levels are low, your body may tap into these reserves to correct the problem.
Manganese • Helps form bones • Helps metabolize amino acids, cholesterol, and carbohydrates	AI M: 2.3 mg W: 1.8 mg	11 mg	Pineapple, nuts, whole grains, legumes, spinach, sweet potatoes, tea	If you take supplements or have manganese in your drinking water, be careful not to exceed the upper limit. Those with liver damage or whose diets supply abundant manganese should be especially vigilant.
Molybdenum • Part of several enzymes, one of which helps ward off a form of severe neurological damage in infants	RDA 45 mcg	2,000 mcg	Organ meats, whole grains, green leafy vegetables, milk, beans	Molybdenum deficiencies are rare.
Phosphorus • Helps build and protect bones and teeth • Part of DNA and RNA • Helps convert food into energy • Part of phospholipids, which carry lipids in blood and help shuttle nutrients into and out of cells	RDA 700 mg	Ages 19 to 70: 4,000 mg Ages 71+: 3,000 mg	Salmon, yogurt, milk, halibut, turkey, chicken, beef, lentils, almonds, cheese, peanuts, eggs, whole-grain bread, carbonated cola	Phosphorus deficiencies are rare. Certain drugs (including some diuretics, ACE inhibitors, and antacids) bind with phosphorus, making it unavailable and causing bone loss, weakness, and pain.
Potassium • Balances fluids in the body • Helps maintain steady heartbeat and send nerve impulses • Needed for muscle contractions • May lower blood pressure • May benefit bones	AI 4,700 mg	Not known	Apricots, lentils, prunes, squash, raisins, potatoes, kidney beans, orange juice, soybeans, bananas, milk, spinach	Food sources do not cause toxicity, but high-dose supplements might. Those with type 1 diabetes and those taking certain drugs—such as ACE inhibitors, certain diuretics, or nonsteroidal anti-inflammatory drugs—should speak with their doctor before increasing potassium intake.

continued

Table 2 *continued*

MINERAL AND BENEFITS	RDA OR AI*	UL*	GOOD FOOD SOURCES (listed most to least)	DID YOU KNOW?
Selenium • Acts as an antioxidant, neutralizing unstable molecules that damage cells • Helps regulate thyroid hormone activity	RDA 55 mcg	400 mcg	Brazil nuts, tuna, halibut, sardines, ham, shrimp, pasta, beef steak, turkey, beef liver, chicken, cottage cheese, brown rice, eggs, fortified cereals, whole-wheat bread, oatmeal, spinach, milk, yogurt	A single 1-ounce serving of Brazil nuts can contain almost twice the RDA of selenium.
Sodium • Balances fluids in the body • Helps send nerve impulses • Needed for muscle contractions • Influences blood pressure; even modest reductions in sodium consumption can lower blood pressure	AI Ages 19 to 50: 1,500 mg Ages 51 to 70: 1,300 mg Ages 71+: 1,200 mg	2,300 mg	Salt, soy sauce, processed foods such as cereals, bread, hot dogs, cheese spreads, tomato juice, canned soups, macaroni and cheese, corned beef hash, pretzels, ham, potato chips, sunflower seeds	While experts recommend that people limit sodium intake to 2,300 mg, Americans typically report consuming 2,300 to 4,700 mg a day (and the real total may be higher, as this does not include salt added at the table). The 2,300-mg upper limit is roughly equivalent to the amount of sodium in 1 teaspoon of table salt.
Zinc • Required for making proteins and DNA • Supports immune system function	RDA M: 11 mg W: 8 mg	40 mg	Oysters, beef, crab, fortified cereals, lobster, pork chops, baked beans, chicken, yogurt, cashews	Zinc lozenges may shorten the duration of the common cold.

*RDA = Recommended Dietary Allowance; AI = adequate intake; UL = tolerable upper intake level.

NOTE: Sulfur is considered a major mineral, but there is no formal RDA, DV, AI, or UL for it. Therefore, we have not included it in the table.

Making sense of scientific studies

Even the most promising finding about a vitamin or mineral must work its way through a hierarchy of studies before scientists can draw firm conclusions about it. It's wise to read carefully and consider the weight of the evidence before you rush off in search of the latest supplement to garner headlines. When it comes to diet and nutrition, each type of study faces a special set of challenges and limitations.

Laboratory studies are done in test tubes or animals. They can suggest how and why a vitamin, mineral, or phytochemical might work, but the findings don't automatically translate to the human body.

Observational studies (also called epidemiological studies) are done in large populations of people—sometimes 100,000 or more—and can run for decades. Scientists collect data at regular intervals. By comparing people who stay healthy with those who fall ill, researchers try to identify factors that could account for the differences. Such studies can be very powerful, since they follow what people actually do in their lives over many years. But they cannot prove cause and effect, only correlations. For example, people who eat blueberries might be healthier because they live healthier lives in general, not because they eat blueberries. Scientists try to adjust for such "confounding" factors, but still cannot draw firm conclusions. Both types of observational studies have limitations:

- **Case-control studies** first identify people with a particular condition ("cases"), then select similar people who don't have that condition ("controls"), and ask everyone about factors in the past that may be related to the condition. These studies may be tainted by problems called "selection bias" (when cases aren't similar enough to the controls) or "recall bias" (when people remember things differently from how they actually happened).
- **Cohort studies** (such as the Nurses' Health Study) begin when researchers identify a large group of people who are initially free of a particular condition, ask about current risk factors, and then follow participants over time to see who develops the condition and who does not. Because participants are routinely questioned about their diet and lifestyle *before* developing the condition, cohort studies are a stronger observational design. However, they often rely on self-reports on dietary questionnaires—which can be subjective and less accurate.

Metabolic studies typically involve a small number of volunteers who eat specially prepared meals for short time periods. These studies are rigorous and closely controlled, but are too brief to show actual effects on disease over the long term. Instead, researchers use them to track changes in risk factors, such as high blood pressure or cholesterol.

Randomized controlled trials are typically considered the gold standard. The researchers randomly assign people to receive either an active treatment (such as a vitamin or mineral supplement) or a placebo (which looks the same, but is inactive). These studies can directly test whether the treatment makes a difference. However, they may be too short to observe long-term consequences. Also, if participants do not stay with the assigned treatment, findings could be blurred or even eradicated. Lastly, these studies may involve participants who are in better or worse health than you are, so they may not yield information that is relevant to you.

Meta-analysis is a statistical strategy that identifies previously published studies containing comparable data and assesses all the evidence together, looking for patterns—in effect, it's a study of studies. A key strength of meta-analysis is the ability to combine data from multiple previously published studies. A potential limitation is that the reliability of the final estimate depends almost entirely on the quality of the individual studies that go into the meta-analysis. Further, when very different studies are combined, the result may be harder to interpret and generalize. ▼

Cast of characters: From vitamin A to zinc

This chapter features a broad overview of the best-known vitamins and minerals. For each nutrient described here, you'll find the following information:

- The Recommended Dietary Allowance (RDA) or adequate intake (AI) for people ages 19 and older (with sex and age differences noted when applicable) and a brief description of the nutrient's role in the body.
- A summary of the data linking the nutrient to protection against various health problems. If a condition is not listed, that means there is insufficient evidence to support a connection.
- Recommendations about taking the nutrient in supplement form.
- A table of selected food sources containing the nutrient, with an emphasis on the best sources in commonly consumed foods. For more information, you can also search the U.S. Department of Agriculture (USDA) National Nutrient Database for Standard Reference exhaustive lists of foods organized by nutrient content. (There is a shortcut to it at www.health.harvard.edu/foodsearch.)

As a rule, your best strategy is to get vitamins and minerals from foods, not supplements. A vast amount of research has shown that you can cut your risk for chronic disease and disability by following a healthy diet, as well as by exercising regularly, maintaining a healthy weight, and not smoking. The evidence for taking high-dose, individual vitamin and mineral supplements is much less convincing. If you're worried about lung cancer, for example, quitting smoking will have a much greater impact on your health than taking supplements.

Before taking a supplement that delivers more than the recommended daily amount of any nutrient, discuss your decision with your doctor. Your medical history, genetic profile, and medications may affect the doses and types of supplements you can safely take.

Vitamin A and carotenoids

RDA for men: 3,000 IU (900 mcg)
RDA for women: 2,333 IU (700 mcg)

"Eat your carrots, they're good for your eyes!" This oft-heard advice is rooted in truth: carrots are rich in beta carotene, which can be converted in the body into vitamin A. The most usable form of vitamin A, retinol, is essential to the proper function of the retina, the light-sensitive tissue lining the back of the eye. But that's only one reason you need vitamin A (and should eat your carrots). In addition to its role in healthy vision, vitamin A aids bone growth and helps regulate the body's infection-fighting abilities.

Some of your vitamin A comes from compounds like beta carotene that convert to vitamin A in the body. But most adults get far more of their vitamin A from animal-based foods, including liver, milk, and eggs, which contain preformed vitamin A. In addition, most fat-free milk and dried nonfat milk solids are fortified with vitamin A to replace the amount lost when the fat is removed. Many breakfast cereals are vitamin A–fortified as well. According to the National Health and Nutrition Examination Survey, a long-running study of the health status of Americans, men and women get slightly less than the amounts recommended, but enough to serve their body's needs.

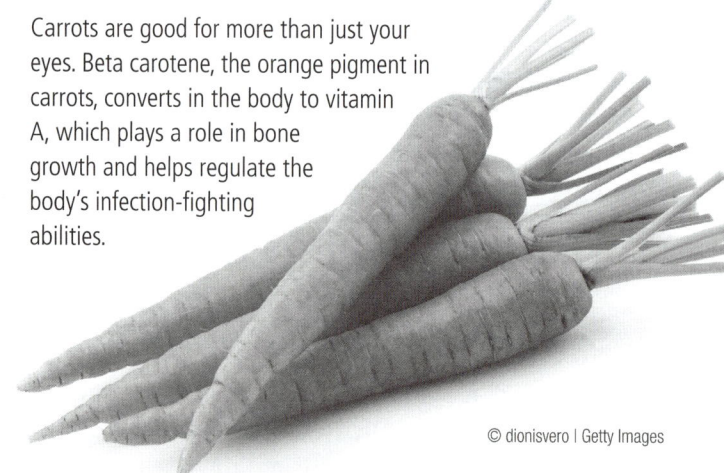

Carrots are good for more than just your eyes. Beta carotene, the orange pigment in carrots, converts in the body to vitamin A, which plays a role in bone growth and helps regulate the body's infection-fighting abilities.

Because vitamin A is a fat-soluble vitamin that's stored in the body, it is possible to build up toxic levels if you consume too much. It's much less likely that you'll overdose on beta carotene, since the body slows down its conversion to vitamin A when it already has enough.

Beta carotene is not the only natural substance that the body can convert to vitamin A. It is just one in a large family of compounds known as carotenoids. Found in many fruits and vegetables, carotenoids are yellow, orange, and red pigments that make carrots orange, for example, and tomatoes red. Although more than 600 carotenoids have been identified, most nutrition research has focused on alpha carotene, beta carotene, lycopene, lutein, zeaxanthin, and beta cryptoxanthin. The carotenoids may contribute to health in multiple ways. Alpha carotene and beta cryptoxanthin, for example, can be converted to vitamin A in the body, just like beta carotene. These are called provitamin A carotenoids. Many of the carotenoids also appear to function as antioxidants.

People in the United States obtain one-quarter to one-third of their vitamin A from carotenoids—most commonly from carrots, cantaloupe, sweet potatoes, and spinach. There is no RDA for beta carotene or other carotenoids, but 3 mg to 6 mg daily is enough to keep blood levels in a range linked to a lower risk of chronic disease, according to the Health and Medicine Division.

Cancer

Epidemiological studies suggest that people who eat foods rich in beta carotene and vitamin A are less likely to develop many types of cancer, especially lung cancer.

That said, when researchers tested beta carotene supplements in smokers, they found that people who took the supplements were *more* likely to develop lung cancer. In one study, heavy smokers who took 30 mg of beta carotene plus 25,000 IU (7,500 mcg) of vitamin A daily were 46% more likely to die of lung cancer than those taking a placebo. Subsequent randomized clinical trials of predominantly nonsmoking men and women have not replicated this finding, but instead found that taking supplements presented neither benefit nor risk for total and specific types of cancer. Experts now advise people—especially former and current smokers—not to take beta carotene supplements for cancer prevention.

Cardiovascular disease

Beta carotene supplements have no long-term effects on the development of cardiovascular disease. In the Physicians' Health Study, involving 22,071 male physicians in the United States, half were given beta carotene supplements and half were not. After 12 years of supplementation, no differences between the two groups—positive or negative—emerged in regard to heart attack, stroke, cancer, or death from all causes. A two-year study of the effects of beta carotene supplementation on 39,876 women, who were healthy at the start of the trial, also found no benefit or harm in terms of cardiovascular disease, cancer, or death.

Eye diseases

Healthy eyes depend on vitamin A as well as carotenoids that aren't transformed into vitamin A. Lutein and zeaxanthin are the only carotenoids found in the retina, the light-sensing layer of cells in the back of the eye. Intake of spinach and kale, two lutein-rich vegetables, appears to moderately reduce the risk of cataracts (the clouding of the normally clear lens of the eye). And one study found that women who got the most lutein and zeaxanthin through their diets lowered their risk of needing surgery to remove a cataract by 22% compared with women who got the least.

Evidence from the Age-Related Eye Disease Study (AREDS) and a follow-up study called AREDS2 suggest that beta carotene and lutein-zeaxanthin supplements can also prevent or slow age-related macular degenera-

Selected food sources of vitamin A and beta carotene*

FOOD	INTERNATIONAL UNITS (IU)
Sweet potato, baked in skin, 1 large	34,592
Beef liver, pan fried, 3 ounces	22,175
Carrots, raw, chopped, 1 cup	21,384
Spinach, frozen, boiled, ½ cup	11,458
Cantaloupe, raw, balls, 1 cup	5,986
Milk, nonfat, 1 cup, fortified	500

*Animal sources contain preformed vitamin A; plant sources contain beta carotene.
Source: USDA National Nutrient Database for Standard Reference.

tion (AMD), a condition that leads to blurred, distorted sight and blind spots in the field of vision. In the first AREDS trial, researchers tested a formulation consisting of vitamin C (500 mg), vitamin E (400 IU), beta carotene (15 mg), copper (2 mg), and zinc (80 mg) in 3,640 people ages 55 to 80 years old with varying stages of AMD. (Copper was added to the mix because high levels of zinc may cause copper deficiency.)

While not a cure, the formulation slowed progression to advanced AMD by about 25%. A slightly altered formulation was tested in the AREDS2 trial. Given the increased risk of lung cancer found among smokers and former smokers who took beta carotene supplements, the researchers removed beta carotene and replaced it with a combination of lutein (10 mg) and zeaxanthin (2 mg). They also added omega-3 fatty acids (1,000 mg) to the mix. This time, the results showed that lutein and zeaxanthin were a safe and effective alternative to beta carotene for AMD, but there was no effect of omega-3s on eye health. In addition, neither of the formulations tested in the AREDS trials reduced the risk of developing cataracts.

Recommendations

- If you take a multivitamin, make sure most or all of the vitamin A comes in the form of beta carotene and not retinol or retinyl compounds (the preformed versions of vitamin A). These can be toxic at high levels.
- If you are taking a multivitamin to improve your eye health, look for a formulation that contains amounts of vitamins C and E, zinc, copper, lutein, and zeaxanthin similar to those found in the AREDS2 formulation.
- Recommendations from the U.S. Preventive Services Task Force advise against the use of beta carotene supplements to prevent either cardiovascular disease or cancer.

B vitamins

The B vitamins (see "The B list," below left) perform a wide range of important functions throughout the body, such as helping to convert food into energy and maintain the immune system, healthy skin, blood cells, the brain, and the nervous system. Many Americans, especially the elderly, don't meet the RDAs for three of the Bs—B_6, B_{12}, and folic acid. These Bs have garnered the most attention from public health officials and researchers, so we, too, will zero in on them.

Vitamin B_6 (pyridoxine)

RDA, ages 19 to 50: 1.3 mg
RDA for men, ages 51 and older: 1.7 mg
RDA for women, ages 51 and older: 1.5 mg

Your body needs vitamin B_6 to break down protein and build red blood cells. This vitamin occurs naturally in a variety of foods, including meat, poultry,

▶ The B list

The B vitamins consist of eight distinct vitamins that help cells function optimally:

- vitamin B_1: thiamin
- vitamin B_2: riboflavin
- vitamin B_3: niacin or nicotinic acid
- vitamin B_5: pantothenic acid
- vitamin B_6: pyridoxal, pyridoxine, pyridoxamine
- vitamin B_7: biotin
- vitamin B_9: folate, folic acid
- vitamin B_{12}: various cobalamins; commonly cyanocobalamin in vitamin supplements.

Missing from the list above are B_4, B_8, B_{10}, and B_{11}, which were once thought to be important to human health, but were later discovered to be nonessential to humans. Therefore, they are no longer considered vitamins.

Selected food sources of vitamin B_6

FOOD	MILLIGRAMS (MG)
Chickpeas, canned, 1 cup	1.1
Beef liver, pan fried, 3 ounces	0.9
Tuna, yellowfin, fresh, cooked, 3 ounces	0.9
Salmon, sockeye, cooked, 3 ounces	0.6
Chicken breast, roasted, 3 ounces	0.5
Breakfast cereal, fortified with 25% of the DV for vitamin B_6, 1 serving	0.5
Banana, 1 medium	0.4

Source: USDA National Nutrient Database for Standard Reference.

fish, and some fruits and vegetables, and is added to some fortified cereals. Most younger people meet the RDA for B6, but one survey showed that many people over 60 don't: men got 1.2 mg daily instead of the recommended 1.7 mg, and women got 1.0 mg daily instead of 1.5 mg.

Folic acid (vitamin B9, folate)

RDA: 400 mcg

Folic acid or folate (the terms refer, respectively, to the vitamin's synthetic and natural forms) plays a role in the synthesis, repair, and function of DNA, the genetic material found in all cells. Beef liver, leafy green vegetables, and dried beans are good sources. Some Americans, including a fair number of women of childbearing age, don't get enough of this vitamin. That's worrisome, because having insufficient levels just before and during the early stages of pregnancy increases the risk of having a baby with a neural tube defect—a serious malformation of the spine, skull, or brain, such as spina bifida or anencephaly. To address this problem, folic acid has been added to breads, cereals, flours, cornmeal, pastas, rice, and other grain products since 1998, when an FDA regulation mandating the addition took effect. As a result, the average daily intake of folic acid has risen by an estimated 100 micrograms (mcg), and the incidence of neural tube defects has fallen by 25% to 50% in the United States and other countries that require folic acid fortification (although other factors, such as ultrasound screening, may have contributed to the drop as well).

Vitamin B12 (cyanocobalamin)

RDA: 2.4 mcg

Vitamin B12, which is required for proper brain function and a host of chemical reactions within the body, is found naturally only in animal foods (fish, meat, poultry, eggs, and milk). Many fortified cereals contain a synthetic form. Vegans, who avoid all animal-based foods, need to ensure they get enough of this vitamin through fortified foods or supplements. About 6% of people ages 60 and older are deficient in vitamin B12, and nearly one in five is borderline deficient. As you age, it often becomes harder to absorb enough B12 from food. This problem usually reflects reduced production of stomach acid, which liberates B12 from food. But since this stomach acid isn't needed for your body to absorb B12 from supplements or fortified foods, you can avoid a deficiency by getting enough B12 from these sources. A B12 deficiency can cause pernicious anemia (see Figure 3, page 20). This condition is usually treated with monthly injections of B12.

Heart disease

Starting in the mid-1980s, numerous studies noted a link between an increased risk of cardiovascular disease and high blood levels of homocysteine (an amino acid associated with inflammation of blood vessels, including those that feed the heart and brain). Many people with high homocysteine levels are deficient in vitamins B6, B12, and folic acid. Supplements with these vitamins can reduce homocysteine levels within weeks. But this has no effect on the number of heart attacks or deaths from heart disease, according to two

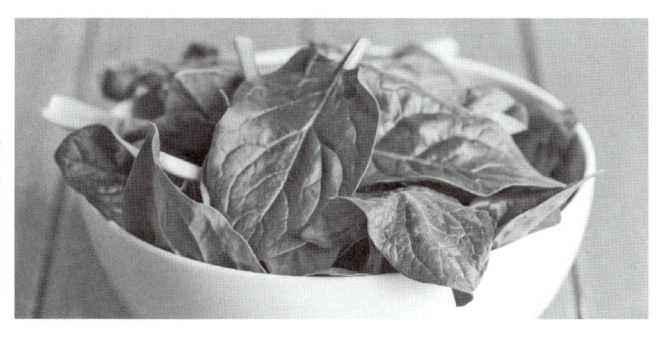

Selected food sources of folic acid

FOOD	MICROGRAMS (MCG)
Beef liver, braised, 3 ounces	215
Spinach, boiled, ½ cup	131
Black-eyed peas (cowpeas), boiled, ½ cup	105
Breakfast cereal, fortified with 25% of the DV for folic acid, 1 serving	100
Rice, white, medium-grain, cooked, ½ cup	90
Asparagus, boiled, 4 spears	89
Spaghetti, enriched, cooked, ½ cup	83
Brussels sprouts, frozen, boiled, ½ cup	78

Source: USDA National Nutrient Database for Standard Reference.

long-term, randomized clinical trials—the Heart Outcomes Prevention Evaluation–2 (HOPE-2) study and the Women's Antioxidant and Folic Acid Cardiovascular Study (WAFACS)—of people at high risk for or with established cardiovascular disease.

Cancer

The relationship between cancer and B vitamins—folic acid, in particular—has proved complex. There's evidence that people with low blood levels of folate are more prone to cancer, and several large, long-term studies suggest that people who consume more folic acid are less likely to develop colon cancer. Other research suggests that greater consumption of folic acid can lower breast cancer risk, at least among women who drink alcohol and have low folic acid levels.

But while adequate amounts of folic acid appear to stifle the formation and spread of early tumors, it's possible that too much may speed up the growth of existing tumors. In fact, one randomized trial found that folic acid supplements increased the recurrence of adenomatous polyps, which can turn into colon cancer. Several studies suggest that excess folic acid may raise the risk of cancer of the colon, breast, and prostate. A study that reviewed cancer registries in the United States and Canada (which also began folic acid fortification in 1998) revealed a slight uptick in colon cancer rates in the early fortification years, when average blood levels of folate doubled. However, the overall steady decline in deaths from colon cancer before and after folic acid fortification suggests that improved screening from colonoscopies is a more likely explanation for the upward blip.

Memory problems

Several epidemiological studies have shown that blood concentrations of vitamins B_6, B_{12}, and folic acid are linked to people's performance on tests of memory and abstract thinking. In one, investigators collected blood from 816 older people. After about four years, 112 of them

Figure 3: B_{12} deficiency and anemia

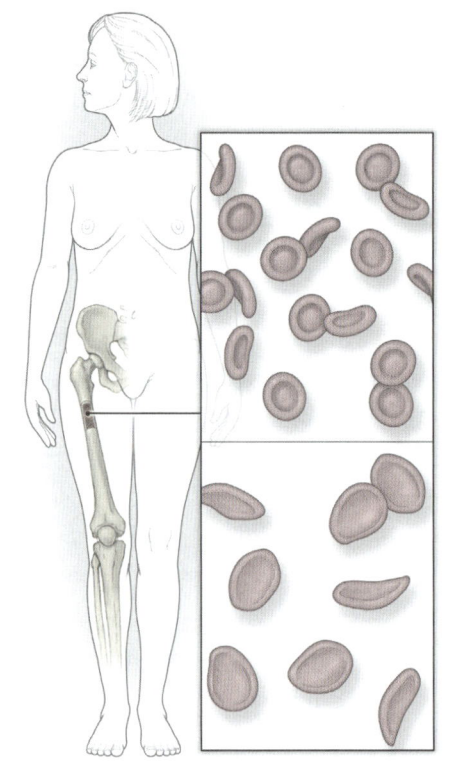

Normal red blood cells

Pernicious anemia

In rare cases, low vitamin B_{12} levels can cause pernicious anemia, a condition in which the bone marrow produces red blood cells that are both larger and less numerous than normal. Symptoms can include yellowish skin, fatigue, shortness of breath, and headaches. Numbness or tingling in the hands and feet and trouble keeping balance are common. Confusion, depression, and memory loss can also occur and are sometimes chalked up to Alzheimer's disease.

Selected food sources of vitamin B_{12}

FOOD	MICROGRAMS (MCG)
Clams, cooked, 3 ounces	84.1
Beef liver, cooked, 3 ounces	70.7
Breakfast cereal, fortified with 100% of the DV for vitamin B_{12}, 1 serving	6.0
Trout, rainbow, wild, cooked, 3 ounces	5.4
Salmon, sockeye, cooked, 3 ounces	4.8
Tuna fish, light, canned in water, 3 ounces	2.5
Cheeseburger, double patty and bun, 1 sandwich	2.1
Milk, low-fat, 1 cup	1.2

Source: USDA National Nutrient Database for Standard Reference.

> ### B bonanza: Boon or bust?
>
> Presumably because of their role in helping cells use energy, B vitamins are often added to energy drinks and nutrition bars—sometimes in extremely high amounts. A can of Red Bull, for example, contains 250% of the Daily Value* (DV) for vitamin B6. And a single 2-ounce bottle of 5-Hour Energy includes a whopping 2,000% of the DV for vitamin B6 and 8,333% of the DV for vitamin B12—and the label even suggests you can drink two bottles per day. Various brands of bottled water, such as Vitaminwater, contain up to four B vitamins in amounts approaching 100% of the DV.
>
> And you can't necessarily trust the labels. According to ConsumerLab.com, which does independent reviews of vitamins and other supplements and related products, one brand of vitamin water the agency tested contained 15 times its claimed amount of folic acid. (Because vitamins degrade over time, manufacturers often include extra in packaged products—but not typically that much more.)
>
> These megadoses do nothing to enhance any bodily functions, and because B vitamins are water-soluble, they're not stored in the body, so any extra is excreted in the urine.
>
> *As described on Nutrition Facts panels, percent Daily Values are based on a 2,000-calorie diet. Your needs may be higher or lower depending on your body size and activity level.

had developed dementia, including 70 diagnosed with Alzheimer's disease. Those who started with higher concentrations of folate were less likely to have suffered cognitive decline. Some small randomized controlled trials also suggest that treatment with folic acid and other B vitamin supplements may slow cognitive decline in older people, perhaps through the B vitamins' ability to lower homocysteine (see "Heart disease," page 19).

That said, a randomized controlled trial of people with mild to moderate Alzheimer's disease found that taking high-dose vitamin B supplements did not slow cognitive decline. And three studies reviewed by the Cochrane Collaboration, an international group of independent experts, did not show any ability of these B vitamins to protect thinking skills or slow age-related decline in healthy older people.

Recommendations

- For most people, the best source of RDA-appropriate levels of B vitamins is a reasonably balanced diet, combined with a multivitamin-multimineral supplement as needed (if there are broader concerns about an overall healthy diet). Be wary of energy drinks and bars that may provide more B vitamins than necessary (see "B bonanza: Boon or bust?" at left).
- **B6:** Avoid supplements that contain more than the RDA for this vitamin, as excess amounts can cause nerve damage. Though the excess will eventually be excreted, the damaging threshold varies from one individual to the next, and before being excreted, the excess can cause damage.
- **Folic acid:** Beware of getting too much of this micronutrient from supplements and fortified foods. Most multivitamins contain 400 mcg, but many fortified breakfast cereals also contain that much. Add a few other enriched grain products (10 pretzels adds 172 mcg, and a cup of spaghetti, 166 mcg) and you're over your daily limit. If you take a daily multivitamin, avoid foods fortified with 300 to 400 mcg of folic acid.
- **B12:** Vegans, who avoid all animal-based foods, and elderly people, who may have trouble absorbing vitamin B12 from food, should consider eating a vitamin B12–fortified breakfast cereal or taking a supplement.

Vitamin C

RDA for men: 90 mg
RDA for women: 75 mg
Smokers: add 35 mg

Vitamin C is perhaps best known for its onetime reputation for preventing and treating the common cold—an idea first promoted in the 1970s by Nobel laureate Linus Pauling. But according to a meta-analysis of 30 placebo-controlled trials, taking up to 2 grams of vitamin C per day does not decrease your chances of catching a cold, although it may very slightly shorten the duration of your sniffles. Many experts who insist on the cold-defying power of vitamin C state that even higher amounts are needed to achieve this effect. However, so far there is no evidence from randomized clinical trials to support this assertion.

In the body, vitamin C is crucial for making collagen, which lends structural support to tendons, ligaments, bones, and blood vessels. This vitamin is also considered to be a potent antioxidant, which is why smokers, who are exposed to more free radicals because of their habit, are advised to consume extra vitamin C.

Most people meet the RDA for vitamin C via their diets. Citrus fruits are rich in vitamin C, but a half cup of sweet red peppers contains roughly a third more than a medium-sized orange.

Heart disease and cancer

Despite a handful of studies hinting that vitamin C might ward off heart disease and cancer, the evidence offers no support for supplemental C. The Physicians' Health Study II, which followed 14,641 men who took 500 mg of vitamin C daily for a decade, found no difference in the number of heart attacks, strokes, or deaths from cardiovascular disease compared with men who took placebos. Results were similar in the Women's Antioxidant Cardiovascular Study (WACS), which included 8,171 female health professionals with a history of cardiovascular disease or several risk factors for the disease: taking 500 mg of vitamin C a day, along with 600 IU of vitamin E and 50 mg of beta carotene every other day, did not reduce the incidence of cardiovascular events over nine years of follow-up. In a separate analysis from the Physicians' Health Study II, researchers found that the likelihood of developing cancer was also nearly identical whether the men took vitamin C or a placebo.

That said, vitamin C supplements might have a modest effect on blood pressure, according to a meta-analysis of data from 29 small randomized, controlled trials that compared vitamin C against a placebo. Researchers found that people who were given a median dose of 500 mg per day of supplemental vitamin C had a drop in systolic blood pressure of 3.8 millimeters of mercury (mm Hg) over the short term. Among participants who had a diagnosis of high blood pressure (hypertension), the drop was greater, at nearly 5 mm Hg.

Eye diseases

Eye tissue contains large amounts of vitamin C, and some studies suggest that the vitamin may help ward off cataracts, which cloud the eye's lens and diminish vision. For instance, one study found that people who consume about eight to 10 times the RDA of vitamin C, through both foods and supplements, were less likely to develop cataracts than people who consumed the RDA. But prospective, randomized clinical trials of more than 35,000 female health professionals and 11,545 male physicians found no association between vitamin C intake and the incidence of cataracts. In a Swedish prospective study that followed more than 24,000 women for about eight years, researchers found that women who took 1,000 mg of vitamin C supplements on a regular basis were actually *more* likely to develop cataracts. In women ages 65 and older, the risk was 38% more than that of women who didn't take vitamin C supplements.

The trial of male physicians also found that taking a daily vitamin C supplement for eight years had no effect—good or bad—on the risk of AMD.

Recommendation

- Taking vitamin C supplements in amounts far higher than the RDA offers no apparent health benefits but is probably harmless, despite the cataract study noted above.

Selected food sources of vitamin C

FOOD	MILLIGRAMS (MG)
Red sweet pepper, raw, ½ cup	95
Orange juice, ¾ cup	93
Orange, 1 medium	70
Grapefruit juice, ¾ cup	70
Kiwifruit, 1 medium	64
Green sweet pepper, raw, ½ cup	60
Broccoli, cooked, ½ cup	51

Source: USDA National Nutrient Database for Standard Reference.

Vitamin D

RDA, ages 1 to 70: 600 IU (15 mcg)
RDA, ages 71 and older: 800 IU (20 mcg)

This fat-soluble vitamin is unique because its primary natural source is sunlight, not food. In fact, it's found naturally in only a few foods. What's more, fatty fish, the main food source of vitamin D, isn't something most Americans eat daily. Milk, which doesn't naturally contain vitamin D, has been fortified with it since the 1930s to help fill the gap; however, dairy products made from milk (such as cheese and ice cream) aren't typically fortified with vitamin D and contain only small amounts. Some brands of yogurt are fortified, and so are some juices and breakfast cereals. For older adults to meet the RDA of 800 IU, they would have to drink at least a quart of fortified milk per day.

Fortunately, most people don't have to rely on their diets for vitamin D, because exposing your skin to sunshine—more specifically, ultraviolet B (UVB) rays—enables the body to make vitamin D, which is why it's also known as the "sunshine vitamin." But the skin's production of vitamin D depends on a number of factors, only some of which are under your control.

The lowdown on low vitamin D levels

Humans first evolved near the equator in Africa, where the sun shines directly overhead for much of the year. Our ancestors there wore little or no clothing and therefore probably produced tens of thousands of IU of vitamin D each day. Heavy pigmentation protected the deeper layers of their skin from sun-induced damage. As some groups of humans migrated away from the equator, their skin lightened to enable faster vitamin D production in conditions with less direct sunshine.

For centuries, people typically spent plenty of time outdoors during much of the year. But in the last 300 years, more people began working indoors, and in the last 100 years, began riding in cars and greatly reduced their daily time outside. (Not only do cars shield people from the sun, they also contribute to air pollution, which screens out some of the UV radiation that reaches Earth.) In the past few decades, putting on sunscreen has become de rigueur before heading outdoors, and in sharp contrast to the trend favoring the "healthy tan" in the mid-20th century, many Americans now intentionally avoid the sun. That's because they want to prevent skin cancer—a valid concern, given that UV radiation is an established risk factor for most of the estimated 3.5 million skin cancers that occur each year in the United States—but it also lessens the amount of vitamin D produced in the skin. All of these changes mean that some of us may be getting less vitamin D than our bodies need. However, true vitamin D deficiency is far less common in the United States than potential vitamin D insufficiency (see "How much vitamin D do you need?" on page 24).

Factors that affect vitamin D production

Where you live, the season of the year, and the time of day all affect how much sunlight—and how much UVB radiation—reaches your skin. The sun's rays are most direct between 10 a.m. and 3 p.m. However, the farther you live from the equator, the less UVB radiation you receive, and it is UVB that prompts your body to produce vitamin D. People who live north of about 37° latitude (picture an imaginary line extending from San Francisco, Calif., to Richmond, Va.) can't make any vitamin D from sunlight from November to March, even if they were to stay outside all day. This phenomenon has to do with the angle of the sunlight: during

Selected food sources of vitamin D

FOOD	INTERNATIONAL UNITS (IU)
Cod liver oil, 1 tablespoon	1,360
Swordfish, cooked, 3 ounces	566
Salmon (sockeye), cooked, 3 ounces	447
Tuna fish, canned in water, drained, 3 ounces	154
Orange juice, fortified, 1 cup	137
Milk, fortified, 1 cup	115–124
Yogurt, fortified with 20% of the DV for vitamin D, 6 ounces	80
Egg, 1 large	41

Source: USDA National Nutrient Database for Standard Reference.

the winter months, the earth tilts away from the sun, increasing the angle at which the sun's light reaches the earth's surface. When this happens, more UVB radiation is absorbed by the ozone layer, lowering or eliminating the amount that can reach a person's skin.

What's more, your age, your skin color, the amount of exposed skin, and your sunscreen use all influence your production of vitamin D. Any of these factors can combine to limit vitamin D production, which is why a large number of Americans—including half of those ages 65 and older—have relatively low levels of vitamin D.

Forms of vitamin D

Vitamin D comes in two forms: D_3 (cholecalciferol) and D_2 (ergocalciferol). D_3, the form made naturally by the body in response to sunlight, is also the form most often used to fortify milk and other foods, such as breakfast cereals. D_2 is made from plant material. Vitamin supplements contain either D_3 or D_2. If you take supplements, some experts recommend choosing one that contains D_3. However, the IOM report cited in the box below concluded that D_2 is just as effective as D_3 at the recommended dosage levels.

Osteoporosis and fractures

One of vitamin D's most important and best-known roles is to signal the intestines to absorb calcium into the bloodstream. Without sufficient vitamin D, your body will break down bone to get the calcium it needs—no matter how much calcium you consume through food and supplements.

How much vitamin D do you need?

Despite widespread assertions in the popular and scientific press that many Americans are deficient in vitamin D, the term "deficiency" isn't strictly accurate. The official definition of a vitamin deficiency means that specific health problems stem solely from the lack of (or inability to use) a specific nutrient. An actual deficiency of vitamin D results in the bone disease known as rickets, which is rare in the United States.

On the other hand, lower-than-optimal levels of specific vitamins, including vitamin D, may increase your risk of numerous health problems, even though they are not solely responsible for these problems. "Insufficiency" may be a better term for these lower levels.

So far, the most clearly established benefit of vitamin D is that it helps the body absorb calcium and therefore promotes healthy bones. However, a steady drumbeat of studies beginning in the 1980s started to build a case that low blood levels of D were connected with a variety of chronic health problems, leading to claims by a number of researchers that the RDA for D was way too low. The confusion and controversy surrounding optimal vitamin D intake and blood values prompted the U.S. and Canadian governments to request that the Institute of Medicine (IOM, now called the Health and Medicine Division) review the evidence on vitamin D and calcium and update the DRIs.

The long-awaited report, *Dietary Reference Intakes for Calcium and Vitamin D*, was published in 2011. The IOM concluded that evidence for benefits other than improved bone health came from studies that could not be considered reliable and provided often-conflicting results.

Based on the evidence for bone benefits, however, the IOM panel increased the RDA for vitamin D to 600 IU for people up to age 70 and to 800 IU for those over 70. That's a fairly sizable boost over the previous recommendations of 200 IU per day through age 50, 400 IU for ages 51 to 70, and 600 IU for ages over 70. The IOM also raised the safe upper limit of daily intake for most age groups from 2,000 to 4,000 IU.

But ultimately, the amount of vitamin D that makes it into your bloodstream is more important than how much you're consuming. There again controversy reigns. While some people argue for much higher levels, the IOM report concluded that vitamin D blood levels above 20 ng/ml are adequate for maintaining healthy bones, and that most people in the United States have values in that range. Other organizations, including the American Association of Clinical Endocrinologists, assert that values between 30 and 50 ng/ml have potential health benefits beyond bone health, so the issue is still not resolved. However, the IOM report cautioned that exceptionally high levels of vitamin D have not been proven to confer additional benefits and have been linked to health problems, challenging the notion that "more is better."

Most healthy adults without symptoms related to vitamin D deficiency do not need to have their blood levels measured. People who should consider vitamin D testing are those with medical conditions that affect fat absorption (including weight-loss surgery) or people who routinely take anticonvulsant medications, glucocorticoids, or other drugs that interfere with vitamin D activity.

There is evidence supporting the role of vitamin D in helping to prevent osteoporosis, the bone-thinning disease, which increases the risk of broken bones (fractures). One in five people dies within a year of experiencing a hip fracture, which is nearly always the result of a fall. In addition to strengthening bones, vitamin D may help reduce fractures by shoring up muscles, thus reducing the chances of falling. One study, which pooled results from 12 randomized controlled trials involving more than 19,000 people older than 60, found that 700 to 800 IU of supplemental vitamin D daily cut the risk of hip and other nonvertebral fractures by about a quarter, compared with calcium supplementation alone or a placebo.

In 2011, the U.S. Preventive Services Task Force (USPSTF) published a meta-analysis and recommendation on vitamin D and calcium supplements. The analysis concluded that combined supplementation of vitamin D and calcium (300 to 1,100 IU per day of vitamin D and 500 to 1,200 mg per day of calcium)—but not vitamin D supplementation alone—can reduce the risk of fractures in older adults. The effects may be more profound among elderly persons in institutionalized settings. In its recommendations, the task force said that for adults living at home (not in assisted living or nursing homes), there isn't enough evidence to determine if vitamin D with calcium supplements can prevent fractures in men, in women who have yet to go through menopause, or in postmenopausal women.

Muscle weakness and falls

Inadequate vitamin D levels can lead to muscle weakness, and getting enough may improve muscle function. Although the USPSTF had previously recommended vitamin D supplementation in adults over age 65 not living in nursing homes who are at increased risk for falls, a 2018 review of seven trials found evidence in five of the studies that supplementation does not reduce falls or injuries from falls. Hence, the USPSTF is now recommending *against* people 65 and older taking vitamin D supplements—as long as they don't have osteoporosis or a vitamin D deficiency.

High blood pressure and heart disease

A handful of observational studies have suggested that people with low vitamin D levels face a higher risk of high blood pressure, heart disease, and strokes. However, two large randomized controlled trials of vitamin D supplementation at lower doses of 400 IU—including one that was part of the large Women's Health Initiative—showed no benefit in reducing the likelihood of heart disease or stroke. Nor did a review of 46 trials published in *JAMA Internal Medicine* find a blood pressure–lowering effect for vitamin D. Even very large doses (an initial dose of 200,000 IU, followed by 100,000 IU taken orally once a month) failed to reduce cardiovascular risk more than a placebo in a three-year randomized controlled trial published in 2017 in *JAMA Cardiology*. Currently, there is insufficient evidence to conclude that vitamin D supplements can lower the risk of high blood pressure, heart disease, or stroke.

A large study called VITAL (the Vitamin D and Omega-3 Trial) was designed to provide more evidence about the potential value of both vitamin D and omega-3 fatty acid supplements in preventing cancer and cardiovascular disease. The trial, sponsored by the National Institutes of Health, recruited 25,871 participants from across the United States—men over age 50 and women over age 55—who had never had a stroke or been diagnosed with heart disease or cancer. Participants were randomly assigned to take either 2,000 IU of vitamin D, 1,000 mg of fish oil, both supplements, or placebos. Results published in late 2018 showed that neither vitamin D nor fish oil reduced total heart-related deaths (heart attacks plus strokes plus deaths from cardiovascular disease), but the omega-3s did significantly reduce the risk of heart attacks (by 28%), when examined separately.

Cancer

Higher blood levels of vitamin D are linked to a lower risk of colon cancer in observational studies—although most of the differences in blood vitamin D levels were related to sunlight exposure, not dietary intake from food or supplements. Still, a cross-sectional study of 3,121 adults ages 50 and older found that those with the highest vitamin D intakes (more than 645 IU per day) were less likely to have cancerous lesions detected via colonoscopy than those with lower intakes. Likewise, an analysis of 16,618 participants in the National Health and Nutrition Examination Survey found a relationship between vitamin D status and colon cancer, but not other types of cancer.

Randomized trials, however, have yet to find benefits for vitamin D supplementation in relation to cancer risk. For instance, one trial that examined vitamin D and calcium supplementation over four years in relation to the incidence of cancer in older women found the combination didn't significantly lower the risk of cancer. And re-analysis of data from the Vitamin D Assessment (VIDA) trial, which was conducted in New Zealand, also found no protective benefit against cancer from consuming high doses of vitamin D once a month for four years.

As for the potential increase in skin cancers from UVB exposure in an effort to generate vitamin D, some analyses suggest that any increase in skin cancer from adding a small amount of unprotected sun exposure (five to 10 minutes between 10 a.m. and 3 p.m. on some or most days to the arms, legs, or back) would be offset by declines in other forms of cancer. There isn't enough solid evidence to determine the benefits or harms of vitamin D supplementation with respect to cancer, but the USPSTF does not recommend taking vitamin D supplements to prevent cancer. Results from the VITAL trial (see "High blood pressure and heart disease," page 25) found no evidence that vitamin D reduced the incidence of cancer, although it may slightly reduce the risk of dying from cancer.

Recommendations

- When possible, get your vitamin D from foods and from modest sun exposure, making sure to avoid a sunburn. Five to 10 minutes of sun exposure on some or most days of the week to the arms, legs, or back without sunscreen will enable you to make enough of the vitamin. The sun is strongest between 10 a.m. and 3 p.m. If you live north of the 37th parallel, which broadly cuts the country in half horizontally, you can only get adequate sun exposure to make vitamin D during the summer months. If you live south of it, the sun is strong enough for this purpose almost year-round.

- If getting enough sun-generated vitamin D is not feasible and you don't consume much vitamin D in your diet, then consider a daily multivitamin or separate supplement to meet the recommended dietary intake of 600 to 800 IU per day. (Most multivitamins now contain 1,000 IU.).

- If you do take more than 1,000 IU daily in the form of oral supplements, be sure to stay well below the safe upper limit of 4,000 IU. The potential benefits of higher amounts remain controversial.

Vitamin E

RDA: 22 IU (15 mg)

Your body needs vitamin E. It acts as an antioxidant and also plays a role in immune function and blood clotting. But you probably don't need a lot of it. Multiple studies have shown no beneficial effects from vitamin E supplements for heart disease, cancer, or cognitive decline (see "Mind and memory," page 27), making a strong case for avoiding these amber-colored capsules altogether.

Vitamin E exists in eight different chemical forms in plants. Alpha tocopherol is the most biologically active and second most available form of vitamin E in the diet, whereas gamma tocopherol is the most common dietary form of vitamin E but is not as biologically active.

Nuts, seeds, and vegetable oils (as well as salad dressings and margarines made from these oils) are

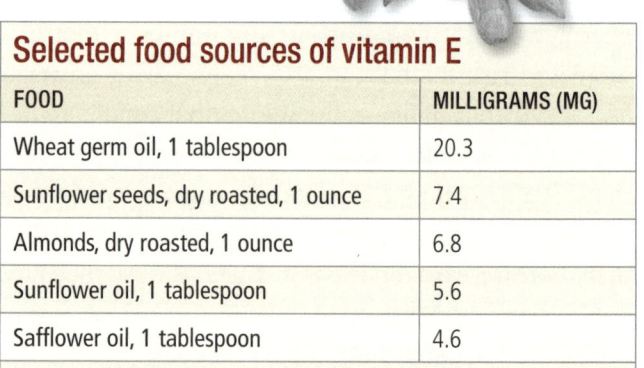

Selected food sources of vitamin E

FOOD	MILLIGRAMS (MG)
Wheat germ oil, 1 tablespoon	20.3
Sunflower seeds, dry roasted, 1 ounce	7.4
Almonds, dry roasted, 1 ounce	6.8
Sunflower oil, 1 tablespoon	5.6
Safflower oil, 1 tablespoon	4.6

Source: USDA National Nutrient Database for Standard Reference.

the best food sources of vitamin E. The National Health and Nutrition Examination Survey suggests that most Americans don't get the RDA for vitamin E, but these estimates likely underestimate actual intake because people typically don't recall how much fat (often vegetable oils) they add during cooking or don't know how much is in the prepared foods they consume.

Heart disease

As is the case with many vitamins, observational studies provided the first suggestion of a potential benefit—in this case, that people with higher vitamin E intakes were less likely to develop heart disease. So, in 1999, the GISSI-Prevenzione randomized trial tested the effects of supplementation, enrolling Italians with recent heart attacks and randomizing them to a vitamin supplement or usual care. No benefits were seen for any outcome, including total deaths or second heart attacks. In 2005, results from the Women's Health Study, a randomized trial that followed about 36,000 women for more than 10 years, showed that an every-other-day supplement of 600 IU of vitamin E did not reduce the risk of having a heart attack or stroke. However, it did decrease the risk of dying from cardiovascular disease by about 25%.

Expectations for vitamin E faded further as the results from other randomized trials came in. A study called HOPE-TOO (the Heart Outcomes Prevention Evaluation—The Ongoing Outcomes) included almost 4,000 people, ages 55 and over, with existing vascular disease or diabetes. Half were randomly selected to take 400 IU of vitamin E daily, and the others to take a placebo. After seven years, vitamin E had not provided any more protection against heart disease or cancer than the placebo. In addition, the vitamin E takers were more likely to have developed heart failure and to have been hospitalized for it.

Another randomized controlled trial, the Physicians' Health Study II, also found no benefit from 400 IU of vitamin E taken every other day for preventing heart disease, stroke, or death from heart disease. In fact, vitamin E appeared to increase the risk of bleeding (hemorrhagic) stroke.

Based on these findings, the USPSTF recommends against taking vitamin E supplements to prevent cardiovascular disease. A large meta-analysis published in 2018 reinforced the notion that vitamin E supplementation is not necessary for cardiovascular disease prevention.

Cancer

Some observational studies have linked higher vitamin E intake with lower risks of breast and prostate cancers, but not consistently. And findings from the Women's Health Study, in which healthy women ages 45 and older took 600 IU of vitamin E or a placebo every other day for 10 years, showed no difference in cancer rates between the two groups.

In October 2008, the National Cancer Institute halted the Selenium and Vitamin E Cancer Prevention Trial (SELECT), which was designed to test whether 200 mcg of selenium and 400 IU of vitamin E, taken alone or in combination, could lower the risk of prostate cancer in nearly 35,000 men. Contrary to expectations, the fewest cases of prostate cancer actually occurred in the placebo group, in which 529 men developed prostate cancer, compared with 575 of those taking selenium alone, 555 of those taking vitamin E plus selenium, and 620 of those taking vitamin E alone. Over all, the daily vitamin E supplement alone significantly *increased* the risk of prostate cancer among these healthy men—which is why the trial was halted early.

For this reason, the USPSTF recommends against taking vitamin E supplements for the purpose of preventing cancer (or cardiovascular disease, as previously stated).

Mind and memory

Despite some promising early suggestions that large amounts of vitamin E might slow the progression of Alzheimer's, results from research have been disappointing. In a study of about 770 people with mild cognitive impairment, often a precursor to Alzheimer's disease, 2,000 IU of vitamin E per day showed no benefit in slowing the advance of the disease compared with a placebo. However, study participants who took vitamin E supplements were able to avoid being institutionalized longer than those who did not. Likewise, a study conducted by the U.S. Department of Veterans Affairs found that among people with mild to moderate Alzheimer's disease, 2,000 IU of vitamin E per day resulted in a slower functional decline compared with placebo.

Eye disorders

People whose diets include about 30 IU of vitamin E daily—double the recommended daily amount—have about a 20% lower risk of developing age-related macular degeneration (AMD), a leading cause of vision loss in people over 60, compared with people who get less than the RDA, according to prospective cohort studies.

The AREDS and AREDS2 studies, which used a 400-IU vitamin E supplement in combination with vitamin C, beta carotene (or lutein and zeaxanthin), zinc, and copper, also found that extra vitamin E may help protect against advanced AMD, slowing its progression by about 25%. However, none of the formulations in either trial tested if it reduced the risk of developing cataracts or stalled their progression. Likewise, in the Physicians' Health Study II, long-term alternate-day use of vitamin E alone or in combination with daily vitamin C had no appreciable benefit or harm on either AMD or cataract risks. And in the SELECT trial, long-term daily supplementation with either vitamin E or selenium alone or in combination did not prevent cataracts.

Recommendations

- Do not take vitamin E supplements unless you have AMD and are taking the vitamin in consultation with your health care provider.
- If you take a multivitamin, make sure it does not contain more than 100 to 200 IU of vitamin E.

Vitamin K

AI for men: 120 mcg
AI for women: 90 mcg

This relatively unknown vitamin got its name from *koagulation*, the German word for coagulation (blood clotting), because vitamin K is essential for that process. Vitamin K also helps produce a key protein used in bone remodeling, and it blocks substances that speed the breakdown of bone. Moreover, it helps regulate calcium excretion from the body in urine.

Vitamin K is found in green leafy vegetables, soybeans, and commonly used cooking oils. People who shy away from salads and other greens may be low in this vitamin. If you take the blood-thinning medication warfarin (Coumadin), it's important to keep your vitamin K intake about the same every day, because the drug interferes with the way vitamin K helps produce clotting proteins. The more vitamin K you consume, the more warfarin you need in order to reach the desired anti-clotting levels.

Fractures

Low vitamin K levels have been linked to a higher risk of hip fractures in at least two epidemiological studies, but other research shows no association between dietary vitamin K and bone mineral density, bone strength, or fracture rates.

Recommendations

- Try to meet your daily requirement for vitamin K from the foods you eat.
- If you take warfarin and a multivitamin, check to see if it contains vitamin K, which is found in some prepa-

Selected food sources of vitamin K

FOOD	MICROGRAMS (MCG)
Collards, frozen, boiled, ½ cup	530
Turnip greens, frozen, boiled, ½ cup	426
Spinach, raw, 1 cup	145
Kale, raw, 1 cup	113
Broccoli, chopped, boiled, ½ cup	110
Soybeans, roasted, ½ cup	43
Edamame, frozen, prepared, ½ cup	21

Source: USDA National Nutrient Database for Standard Reference.

rations in amounts ranging from 10 mcg to 80 mcg. For people who usually get a fair amount of vitamin K from food, the extra vitamin K found in a multivitamin is probably not enough to affect your daily warfarin requirement. But if you get little or no vitamin K in your diet, even a small amount (25 mcg) could upset the balance between vitamin K and warfarin and require a higher daily dose of the drug. Consult your health care provider for more detailed advice.

Calcium

RDA for men, ages 19 to 70: 1,000 mg
RDA for men, ages 71 and older: 1,200 mg
RDA for women, ages 19 to 50: 1,000 mg
RDA for women, ages 51 and older: 1,200 mg

Mention calcium, and most people think of bones. It's true that calcium builds strong bones and teeth, but it also helps muscles to contract, blood to clot, and nerves to send signals to one another.

People who eat a couple of servings of dairy products along with some fruits and vegetables every day probably get close to the RDA of this common mineral. Still, doctors often advise women to take calcium and vitamin D supplements to ward off osteoporosis—the bone-weakening disease that is a common cause of fractures and is far more prevalent among women than men.

The IOM's 2011 report *Dietary Reference Intakes for Calcium and Vitamin D* found that most people get adequate amounts, with the exception of girls ages 9 to 18, who have higher requirements for this mineral. The report also concluded that some postmenopausal women who take calcium supplements to protect against osteoporosis might be getting too much.

Some experts believe that the RDAs for calcium may be higher than necessary, given that very high calcium intakes don't necessarily protect against fractures and may raise the risk of prostate cancer. They also note that in countries such as India, Japan, and Peru, average daily calcium intake is as low as 300 mg per day—yet fractures are far *less* common in those countries than in the United States. However, other important bone health factors, such as higher levels of physical activity and sun exposure (increasing vitamin D formation), could account for the difference.

Selected food sources of calcium

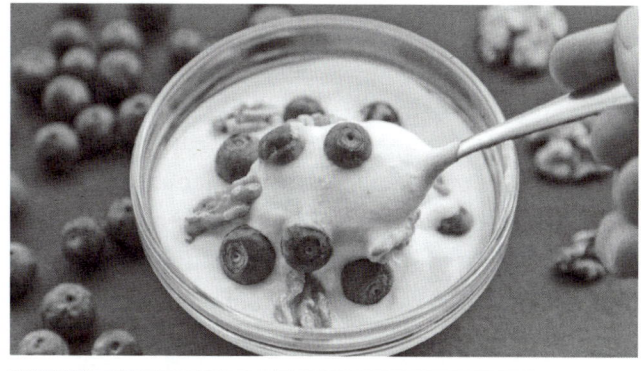

FOOD	MILLIGRAMS (MG)
Yogurt, plain, low-fat, 8 ounces	415
Mozzarella, part skim, 1.5 ounces	333
Milk, nonfat, 8 ounces	299
Soymilk, calcium-fortified, 8 ounces	299
Orange juice, calcium-fortified, 6 ounces	261
Tofu, soft, made with calcium sulfate, ½ cup	138
Turnip greens, fresh, boiled, ½ cup	99

Source: USDA National Nutrient Database for Standard Reference.

The USPSTF has concluded that there is not enough evidence to determine if calcium and vitamin D supplements taken together can prevent bone fractures—and it warns that in older women, they may even lead to kidney stones.

Fractures

Although calcium is clearly important for sturdy bones, evidence that a high calcium intake can prevent fractures isn't as strong you might think. For example, observational results from the Physicians' Health Study and Nurses' Health Study showed that people who drank no more than one glass of milk per week weren't any more likely to break a hip or forearm than were those who drank two or more glasses per week. And a meta-analysis of prospective trials found no association between calcium intake and fracture risk. What's more, the combined results of randomized trials that compared calcium supplements with a placebo showed that calcium supplements did not protect against fractures of the hip or other bones.

Because many people are low in vitamin D, which is crucial for calcium absorption, studies that look at the two nutrients together may be a fairer test. A trial of 36,000 healthy postmenopausal women (conducted as part of the Women's Health Initiative) found that taking calcium and vitamin D supplements cut hip fracture rates by only 12% over all. Yet when researchers analyzed the impact on particular subsets of women, they found that women of any age in the study who consistently took the supplements (as opposed to those who tended to miss doses) had a 29% reduction. The best way to maintain bone strength, however, is to do weight-bearing exercise regularly.

High blood pressure and heart disease

Some research suggests a low calcium intake may contribute to high blood pressure (hypertension), but calcium's exact role is unknown. One theory holds that a lack of calcium in the diet predisposes your body to retain sodium, which raises blood pressure. For this reason, it may be especially important that salt-sensitive people with high blood pressure get enough calcium. (Nearly half of all people with high blood pressure are salt-sensitive, meaning their blood pressure rises in relation to the amount of salt in their diet.)

Efforts to control blood pressure with calcium supplements have had mixed results. Studies found that supplements successfully reduced blood pressure in pregnant women with elevated blood pressure. But clinical trials involving people with essential hypertension (that is, hypertension with no known cause) have been largely disappointing. For most people, calcium supplements either made no difference or reduced blood pressure only slightly—by an average of 1 to 2 millimeters of mercury (mm Hg) in the systolic level (the first and higher number in a blood pressure reading). Although some people experienced larger reductions in blood pressure with the supplements, there seems to be no common denominator, such as race or sex, among those who achieved such improvements.

Most importantly, calcium supplements may be linked to a higher risk of heart attacks in randomized trials. A meta-analysis of nine randomized controlled trials suggested that people who were assigned calcium supplements may have about a 25% higher risk of heart attacks, compared with placebo.

Cancer

Many observational studies show that people whose diets are rich in calcium and dairy products tend to have a lower risk of colon cancer. Less certain are findings that suggest some protective effect against lung and breast cancers. In fact, some observational studies have linked calcium and dairy intake to *higher* risks of ovarian cancer and prostate cancer. For example, data from the Health Professionals Follow-up Study found that men who got more than 2,000 mg of calcium a day were almost three times as likely to develop advanced prostate cancer as men who got less than 500 mg a day. The Nurses' Health Study investigators noted that milk, which is a major source of calcium, might contain another substance that raises ovarian cancer risk. The risk, if it is real, is probably not caused by calcium itself—since calcium supplements seem safe for women—but by the high levels of natural hormones or lactose found in milk.

Kidney stones

The Women's Health Initiative included a randomized clinical trial of calcium and vitamin D supplements among more than 36,000 postmenopausal women ages 50 to 79. Half took daily doses of 1,000 mg of calcium carbonate and 400 IU of vitamin D$_3$, and half took a placebo, for seven years. Among the women taking active pills, 449 developed kidney stones, compared with only 381 in the placebo group.

Recommendations

- Since calcium supplements may increase the risk of heart attacks, kidney stones, and (in men) prostate cancer, try to get adequate calcium from your diet.
- If you aren't meeting the recommended intake of calcium—say, because you don't drink milk or eat other dairy foods—you may want to consider a supplement, although the evidence that this actually prevents fractures is not strong.
- If you take calcium carbonate supplements, which

include antacid pills like Tums and Rolaids, take them just after a meal, since they require stomach acid to be absorbed.
- Calcium citrate isn't as dependent on stomach acid, so it can be taken any time. Calcium citrate is preferred if you take medications that reduce stomach acid (such as Prevacid, Prilosec, Tagamet, or Zantac).
- The body can absorb only about 500 to 600 mg of the mineral at a time, so divide your dose if you take more than that amount.

Magnesium

RDA for men, ages 19 to 30: 400 mg
RDA for men, ages 31 and older: 420 mg
RDA for women, ages 19 to 30: 310 mg
RDA for women, ages 31 and older: 320 mg

If you eat whole-grain bread and your tap water is "hard"—meaning it contains relatively high levels of minerals—you probably consume more magnesium than a person who favors white bread and drinks "soft" water. Why? The refining process used to make white flour strips away the magnesium-rich germ and bran layer of the wheat, along with a number of other nutrients (see Figure 4, above right). And hard water, which is more common in the Midwestern and Southwestern states, contains more magnesium than soft water. Magnesium is also found in nuts, legumes (beans and peas), and seeds, as well as many vegetables.

Selected food sources of magnesium

FOOD	MILLIGRAMS (MG)
Almonds, dry roasted, 1 ounce	80
Spinach, boiled, ½ cup	78
Cashews, dry roasted, 1 ounce	74
Cereal, shredded wheat biscuits, 2 large	61
Soymilk, plain or vanilla, 1 cup	61
Edamame, shelled, cooked, ½ cup	50
Peanut butter, smooth, 2 tablespoons	49

Source: USDA National Nutrient Database for Standard Reference.

Figure 4: The grain drain

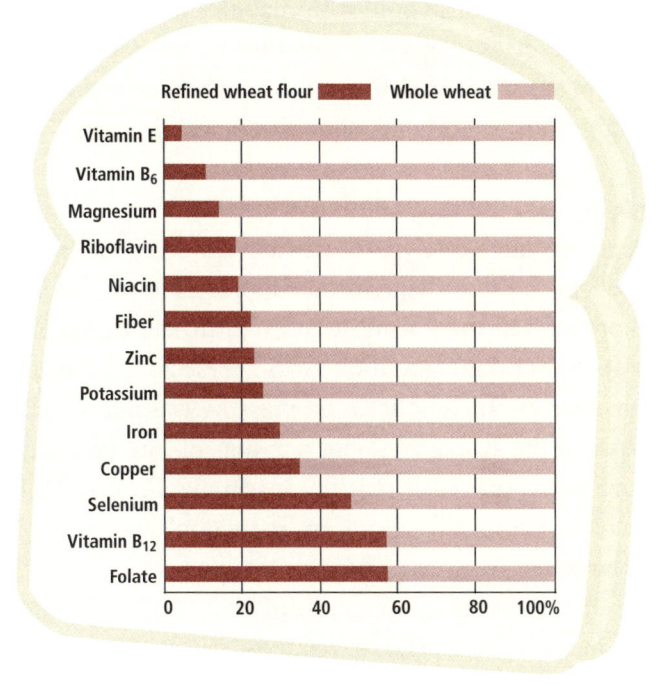

Important nutrients disappear when whole wheat or other grains are refined. As this baker's dozen shows, the losses can be dramatic. For example, refined wheat flour has only 5% of the vitamin E of whole-wheat flour and roughly 10% of the B6.

Many American adults don't get recommended amounts of magnesium, which is key for proper muscle, nerve, and immune function. Magnesium also plays a role in maintaining normal blood pressure and blood sugar.

Diabetes

Magnesium may influence the release and control of insulin, the hormone that regulates blood sugar levels. People with type 2 diabetes (the most common form of the disease) have high blood sugar levels because their bodies have become resistant to insulin or are not producing enough insulin. They also frequently have low magnesium levels. In observational studies such as the Nurses' Health Study and Health Professionals Follow-up Study, researchers found a higher incidence of type 2 diabetes among men and women with low magnesium intakes.

However, small randomized trials of magnesium supplementation have yielded conflicting results. One, which tested high-dose (300-mg) liquid magnesium supplements in people with diabetes and low magnesium levels, suggested the mineral helps improve blood sugar control. But another, which tested even higher doses (600 mg), showed no such benefit.

High blood pressure and heart disease

A recent meta-analysis of 22 randomized controlled trials found that magnesium supplements (in a dose range of 120 to 973 mg per day, with an average of 410 mg per day) can lower blood pressure. The average decrease in systolic blood pressure was 3 to 4 mm Hg, and the average reduction in diastolic blood pressure was 2 to 3 mm Hg. The researchers called it "a small but clinically significant reduction" and worthy of larger-scale investigation.

Blood levels of magnesium that are below the normal range are clearly related to a higher risk of heart electrical disturbances and death. Such levels are typically seen in people with kidney disease or who are taking certain drugs that lower magnesium levels. In a review and meta-analysis of 16 studies, people with a higher level of magnesium circulating in the blood had a 30% lower risk of cardiovascular disease than those with low blood magnesium levels; likewise, people who got adequate magnesium from their diets had a 22% lower risk of suffering from ischemic heart disease (blockages in the heart's arteries that can lead to heart attacks). Higher dietary intake of magnesium has also been associated with a lower risk of sudden cardiac death in women, according to an observational study by Harvard-affiliated scientists. However, more study is needed to determine the role of magnesium in preventing cardiovascular disease and events.

Recommendations

- Try to get sufficient magnesium from healthy foods, such as nuts, spinach, whole grains, and beans. If necessary, consider a multivitamin as a backup source. (Most popular multivitamin brands contain 10% to 30% of the RDA for magnesium.)
- Magnesium supplements should be considered only if your diet contains little to no magnesium; in that case, consult your doctor before starting use.
- Magnesium supplements modestly lower blood pressure, but do not take high doses for this purpose without a doctor's guidance.

Potassium

AI: 4,700 mg

Potassium is necessary for the normal functioning of all cells. It regulates the heartbeat, ensures proper function of the muscles and nerves, and is vital for synthesizing protein and metabolizing carbohydrates.

Thousands of years ago, when humans roamed the earth gathering and hunting, potassium was abundant in the diet, while sodium was scarce. The so-called Paleolithic diet delivered about 16 times more potassium than sodium. Today, most Americans get barely half of the recommended amount of potassium in their diets. The average American diet contains about twice as much sodium as potassium, because of the preponderance of salt hidden in processed or prepared foods, not to mention the dearth of potassium in those foods. This imbalance, which is at odds with how humans evolved, is thought to be a major contributor to high blood pressure, which affects one in three American adults.

Bananas are often touted as

Selected food sources of potassium

FOOD	MILLIGRAMS (MG)
Apricots, dried, ½ cup	1,101
Lentils, cooked, 1 cup	731
Prunes, dried, ½ cup	699
Acorn squash, mashed, 1 cup	644
Raisins, ½ cup	618
Potato, baked, flesh only, 1 medium	610
Orange juice, 1 cup	496
Banana, 1 medium	422
Milk, low-fat, 1 cup	366

Source: USDA National Nutrient Database for Standard Reference.

a good source of potassium, but other fruits (such as apricots, prunes, and orange juice) and vegetables (such as squash and potatoes) also contain this often-neglected nutrient.

High blood pressure

Diets that emphasize greater potassium intake can help keep blood pressure in a healthy range, compared with potassium-poor diets. The DASH trial (Dietary Approaches to Stop Hypertension) compared three regimens. The standard diet, approximating what many Americans eat, contained an average of 3.5 daily servings of fruits and vegetables, which provided 1,700 mg of potassium per day. There were two comparison diets: a fruit- and vegetable-rich diet that included an average of 8.5 daily servings of fruits and vegetables, providing 4,100 mg of potassium per day, and a "combination" diet that included the same 8.5 servings of fruits and vegetables plus low-fat dairy products and reduced sugar and red meat. In people with normal blood pressure, the fruit- and vegetable-rich diet lowered blood pressure by 2.8 mm Hg (in the systolic reading) and 1.1 mm Hg (in the diastolic reading) more than the standard diet. The combination diet lowered blood pressure by 5.5 mm Hg and 3.0 mm Hg more than the standard diet. In people with high blood pressure, the combination diet reduced blood pressure even more, by as much as 11 mm Hg in systolic blood pressure and 5.5 mm Hg in diastolic pressure.

Stroke

High blood pressure is a leading risk factor for strokes, so it's no surprise that higher potassium is also associated with a lower stroke incidence. One prospective study that followed more than 43,000 men for eight years found that men who consumed the highest amounts of dietary potassium (a median of 4,300 mg per day) were 38% less likely to have a stroke as those whose median intake was just 2,400 mg per day. However, a similar prospective study that followed more than 85,000 women for 14 years found a more modest association between potassium intake and the risk of strokes. Additional research has mostly upheld these findings, with the strongest evidence to support high dietary potassium seen in people with high blood pressure and in blacks, who are more prone to high blood pressure than whites.

Recommendations

- Try to eat more produce. Higher potassium consumption from foods, especially fruits and vegetables, may lower blood pressure and the risk of heart disease and strokes.
- Never take potassium supplements without a doctor's prescription, as this can easily cause high blood potassium levels that are dangerous.
- Pay attention to the potassium content of salt substitutes, since it can be high.

Selenium

RDA: 55 mcg

Selenium is a trace mineral known for its antioxidant properties (see "Understanding antioxidants," page 6). It also helps regulate thyroid function and the immune system. Very low intakes cause selenium deficiency, and very high doses cause selenium toxicity. True selenium deficiency and toxicity are rare in the United States, however.

The amount of selenium in foods varies widely, as it depends on the selenium content of the soil where plants are grown or animals are raised. For example, the high plains of northern Nebraska and the Dakotas are rich in selenium, and people living there have the highest selenium intakes in the United States. People who

Selected food sources of selenium

FOOD	MICROGRAMS (MCG)
Brazil nuts, 1 ounce	544
Mixed nuts, oil roasted, without peanuts, salted, 3.5 ounces	421
Tuna, yellowfin, cooked, dry heat, 3 ounces	92
Halibut, cooked, dry heat, 3 ounces	47
Ham, roasted, 3 ounces	42
Cottage cheese, 1% milkfat, 1 cup	20

Source: USDA National Nutrient Database for Standard Reference.

snack on Brazil nuts (found in some canned nut mixtures) may also have high selenium levels, because just an ounce of these nuts contains as much as 10 times the RDA for selenium—a value so high that you shouldn't eat them on a regular basis. Meats, fish, breads, and other nuts are the most common sources of selenium in the American diet, and most people get the RDA.

To determine the degree to which factors beyond diet might influence selenium levels in the body, Harvard researchers examined various factors as they related to selenium measured in toenail clippings, a good biomarker of long-term selenium levels. Cigarette smoking was related to lower selenium levels, with the lowest levels among those who smoked the most cigarettes per day. People with a higher body mass index (BMI) and those living in U.S. states with more selenium in the soil had higher levels.

Cancer

High selenium intakes and high blood levels of selenium are associated with a lower-than-average risk of dying from cancer, including lung, colon, and prostate cancers, according to a handful of observational studies. And people who live in areas of the United States with low soil selenium levels have higher rates of nonmelanoma skin cancer. A study of people with such cancers recruited from dermatology clinics who took 200 mcg of selenium daily found that while the supplement did not affect skin cancer recurrence rates, it did lower the number of cases and deaths from all cancers combined. A 34-year follow-up of a Swedish cohort study called ULSAM found that smokers with low selenium levels at age 50 had higher rates of prostate cancer later in life.

However, the Selenium and Vitamin E Cancer Prevention Trial (SELECT) found no cancer benefits from long-term selenium supplementation. (For more on this trial, see "Vitamin E," page 26.)

Diabetes

In analyses from the SELECT trial and the Nutritional Prevention of Cancer trial, selenium supplements did not reduce the risk of developing diabetes; the SELECT trial even suggested a potential increase in diabetes risk. In contrast, in a large observational analysis in two separate U.S. cohorts, higher selenium levels in toenails (representing higher long-term intake) were linked to a lower risk of diabetes. More research is needed to see whether these conflicting results are due to differences in the dosing, source (dietary selenium versus supplements), underlying population risk, or differences that the study did not measure.

Eye disease

In the eye health analysis report from the SELECT trial, long-term daily supplementation with selenium either alone or in combination with vitamin E did not prevent cataracts.

Recommendation

- There are no known benefits to taking individual selenium supplements. If you want to take supplemental selenium, take it as part of a multivitamin and mineral supplement.

Zinc

RDA for men: 11 mg
RDA for women: 8 mg

Found in cells throughout the body, zinc helps

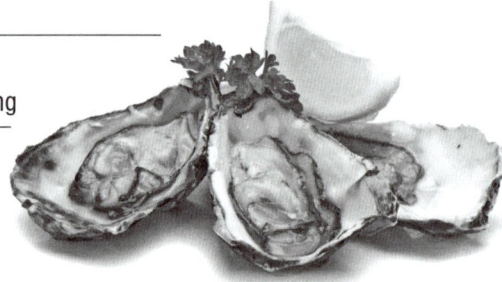

Selected food sources of zinc

FOOD	MILLIGRAMS (MG)
Oysters, cooked, breaded and fried, 3 ounces	74
Beef chuck roast, braised, 3 ounces	7
Crab, Alaskan king, cooked, 3 ounces	6.5
Beef patty, broiled, 3 ounces	5.3
Breakfast cereal, fortified with 25% of the DV for zinc, 1 serving	3.8
Lobster, cooked, 3 ounces	3.4
Pork chop, loin, cooked, 3 ounces	2.9
Baked beans, canned, plain or vegetarian, ½ cup	2.9

Source: USDA National Nutrient Database for Standard Reference.

your immune system fight off bacteria and viruses, which explains why it's been investigated as a potential treatment for the common cold. Your body relies on zinc for wound healing as well as the ability to taste and smell. However, zinc is one of the micronutrients with a small difference between an adequate dose and a harmful one. Most Americans get the RDA for zinc from their diets, since the mineral is found in seafood, meat, fortified cereals, beans, poultry, and dairy products.

The common cold

After a 1984 study concluded that sucking on zinc lozenges could help snuff out the common cold, drug stores began stocking an array of these somewhat odd-tasting lozenges. After 14 double-blind, placebo-controlled trials conducted since the mid-1980s, the result is a draw: half showed that zinc lozenges shortened the duration of a cold, and half showed no effect.

If you decide to use zinc when you get a cold, be aware that following the recommended advice of sucking on a lozenge every two to three hours while you're awake will put you well above 40 mg, the safe upper limit for zinc, as many products contain 13 to 23 mg per lozenge.

There are other potential dangers: high doses of oral zinc can cause gastrointestinal problems or mouth irritation. And there have been several reports of people losing their sense of smell after using zinc nasal gels and sprays.

Cancer

An observational study in older men in Sweden found that high dietary zinc consumption was associated with a lower risk of death from prostate cancer among those men who were diagnosed with this cancer.

Recommendations

- If you try zinc lozenges to shorten the duration of a cold, read the label to be sure you're not taking more than the tolerable upper limit (40 mg a day).
- If you take a multivitamin, don't take an additional zinc supplement. Most already contain the RDA for zinc.

Beyond vitamins: Omega-3s, phytochemicals, and probiotics

We hope that it's clear by now that a well-stocked pantry and refrigerator should be a big part of your first line of defense for staying healthy. Not only do the foods you eat supply essential vitamins and minerals, they also contain many other components that can be beneficial, such as the ones below.

Omega-3 fatty acids

These healthy fats are abundant in certain fatty fish and other seafood. They are also available in much smaller quantities from plant foods and oils, such as walnuts, flaxseed, and canola oil.

The omega-3s have favorable effects on a range of risk factors for heart disease, including blood pressure, heart rate, cholesterol, and inflammation, and they may also help maintain normal heart and blood vessel function. In 1998, data from the Physicians' Health Study showed that men who ate fish once a week were half as likely to die suddenly from a heart attack as men who ate fish less than once a month. One year later, a report in *The Lancet* described a randomized controlled trial in which about 12,000 men who had suffered a heart attack took either a fish oil supplement, 300 mg of vitamin E, both, or neither. Those who took the fish oil supplement had significantly lower rates of heart attack, stroke, or death during the next three-and-a-half years. Sudden death rates dropped by 45%.

People who take statin drugs to lower their cholesterol may also benefit from omega-3 supplements. A randomized trial of 19,000 Japanese men and women with high cholesterol levels found that, after four-and-a-half years, those who took a statin together with an omega-3 supplement had 19% fewer coronary events—in particular unstable angina and nonfatal heart attacks—than those who took the statin alone.

However, a number of meta-analyses of previous observational studies and randomized clinical trials have cast doubt on the value of fish oil supplements, showing insufficient evidence that they reduce the risk of heart attack, heart failure, or stroke in high-risk patients who already have heart disease or specific risk factors. The VITAL trial, released in late 2018 (see "High blood pressure and heart disease," page 25), was the first randomized trial in a "usual risk" population without selected risk factors. Results from the trial showed no significant benefit from fish oil supplements for reducing cancer or deaths from cardiovascular disease, but the trial did find a 28% reduction in heart attack risk. Participants with low fish consumption at the start of the trial (less than 1½ servings per week) appeared to benefit more than others from the omega-3 supplements. According to both the U.S. Dietary Guidelines and the American Heart Association, everyone should try to eat fish, especially oily fish like salmon, sardines, or herring, at least twice a week.

Phytochemicals (bioactives)

Even the most humble fruits and vegetables are replete with phytochemicals—compounds made by plants that affect their flavor, color, scent, and other properties. In recent years, these compounds have also become known as bioactives, because many of them have physiological effects on the human body. The searing bite of hot peppers, the pungent whiff of garlic, the enticing smell of curry, the deep orange hue of carrots, and the red blush on tomatoes all owe a tip of the hat to different phytochemicals.

Although plants develop these compounds for their own purposes, including defense against predators, many of these substances appear to be beneficial for people. The results of certain studies on phytochemicals are now well known—the lutein in dark leafy greens may help protect against specific eye ailments; the lycopene in tomatoes may help defend against prostate disease; the proanthocyanidins in cranberries may help ward off urinary tract infections.

▶ **Beverages in health**

A variety of beverages appear to provide bioactive compounds that are beneficial for health. Coffee contains phytochemicals that are antioxidants and anti-inflammatories, perhaps helping to explain why it's been associated with a reduction in the risk of heart disease, diabetes, and possibly even Alzheimer's disease. Tea contains phytochemicals called catechins that have antioxidant and antimicrobial properties and may fight cancer, heart disease, and infection. Cocoa products contain flavanols that may have benefits for blood pressure, lipid levels, and insulin sensitivity, among other things. Drinks such as kombucha and kefir are plentiful in good bacteria (probiotics) that can boost immunity and digestive health.

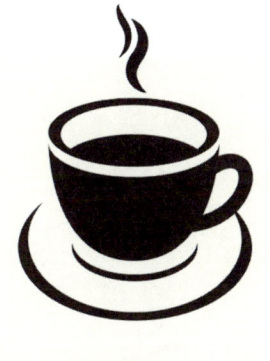

How much of these beverages should you drink to obtain health benefits? That's unclear, but trials are currently ongoing to learn more about their bioactive compounds and health benefits.

Many serve as antioxidants. But there are thousands of phytochemicals in your fruits and vegetables, and in many cases, they work in networks, so taking a few in supplement form is not the best choice. Instead—you guessed it—try to get them from your food (including beverages; see "Beverages in health," above). Here's a bonus: you'll get plenty of vitamins and minerals, too.

Probiotics and prebiotics

Probiotics and prebiotics, along with the gut microbiome (the vast array of good and bad bacteria in your digestive tract), are a hot topic in nutrition these days. Probiotics are good bacteria present in food and supplements. When consumed, they can help bolster populations of good bacteria that have resided in your digestive tract since you were born. Ideally, the good bacteria keep in check the disease-causing bacteria that are also part of your gut microbiome. Initial studies suggest that these good bacteria may help improve your digestion, strengthen your immunity, and suppress inflammation. Prebiotics are primarily the insoluble fibers in foods you eat that feed the good bacteria in your digestive tract.

It's been found that the good bacteria in the gut—which number in the trillions—can be depleted if you eat a lot of sugar, saturated fat, and processed foods (in other words, the typical American diet). Antibiotics also kill large swaths of gut bacteria, both good and bad. And a less diverse, less robust gut microbiome has been associated with certain health conditions such as irritable bowel syndrome (IBS), inflammatory bowel disease, and multiple sclerosis. It's thought that taking probiotics or prebiotics can replenish or diversify these populations.

Probiotics have been best studied for digestive health and IBS, with most studies and meta-analyses showing some benefit from taking supplements. Other preliminary studies have shown benefit for treating seasonal allergies, arthritis, high blood pressure, depression and anxiety, and weight gain.

Food sources are the best way to get probiotics, which are found in fermented foods such as yogurt, kefir, kombucha, miso, tempeh, kimchi, sauerkraut and pickles brined in water and salt, sourdough bread, raw-milk and farmstead cheeses, and aged cheeses such as Swiss, provolone, cheddar, and cottage cheese.

Because you have to eat a lot of these foods to get any purported benefits, a supplement may provide a viable source, although a number of studies have indicated that the bacteria from supplements do not attach well to intestinal walls and therefore do not colonize the gut effectively. If you opt for a supplement, seek a brand containing one or both of the two best studied types, *Lactobacillus* and *Bifidobacterium*. Consumerlab.com, which recently completed a review of probiotic supplements and drinks, advises purchasing a product that contains at least one billion cells per dose. No serious side effects have been noted with the use of probiotics, although if you take too much you may have gas or diarrhea. And if you're allergic to gluten or milk proteins, be aware that many probiotic supplements may contain one or the other.

In comparison to probiotics, it's easier to get prebiotics from foods. They're found in whole-grain products such as oatmeal and whole-grain breads, as well as vegetables like asparagus, leeks, onions, and garlic, and starchy vegetables like sweet potatoes and corn. Beans, lentils, and peas are also good sources. ♥

SPECIAL SECTION

Does your diet deliver the daily recommended dose?

It's easy to look up the daily recommended intake for every vitamin and mineral based on your age and sex. (For vitamins, see Table 1, page 9, and for minerals, see Table 2, page 12, or visit the USDA's website, which you can find at www.health.harvard.edu/DRI.) But how much of each of these nutrients are you actually getting from the foods you eat every day—and do they meet your daily needs?

Focus on food

There are several ways to approach the question of healthy eating. One is to analyze the nutrient content of everything you eat. The other, which we prefer, is to focus on the big picture: eating a balanced diet that contains a variety of colorful fruits and vegetables, whole grains, beans, nuts, dairy products, seafood, lean meats, and poultry. When choosing what to eat, emphasize nutrient-dense foods, which are packed with vitamins and minerals and have relatively few calories (see "Examples of nutrient-dense foods," page 39).

Try the Mediterranean diet

Another approach to getting plenty of vitamins and minerals from food is to use the Mediterranean diet as your guide to healthy eating (see "Mediterranean quiz," below). This eating pattern, with its emphasis on vegetables, fruits, whole grains, olive oil, fish, yogurt, beans, and nuts (plus wine in moderation) provides a wide array of vitamins and minerals. Numerous studies affirm the disease-fighting powers of this approach.

The first U.S.-based study of the diet confirmed that the more closely people followed the Mediterranean eating style, the lower their risk of dying from either heart disease or cancer. The Spanish PREDIMED trial of 7,447 men and women ages 55 to 80 at high risk for cardiovascular disease found that

Mediterranean quiz

How Mediterranean is your diet? Give yourself one point for each "Yes." If you score 6 or higher, you're eating like an Aegean.

	YES	NO
Vegetables (other than potatoes), 4 or more servings a day		
Fruits, 4 or more servings a day		
Whole grains, 2 or more servings a day		
Beans (legumes), 2 or more servings a week		
Nuts, 2 or more servings a week		
Fish, 2 or more servings a week		
Red and processed meat, 1 or fewer servings a day		
Dairy foods, 1 or fewer servings a day		
More unsaturated fat (olive oil and other liquid vegetable oils) than saturated fat (butter, palm oil, bacon fat, etc.)		
TOTAL		

Does your diet deliver the daily recommended dose? | **SPECIAL SECTION**

Examples of nutrient-dense foods

In contrast to potato chips, which contain a lot of calories but not a lot of nutrients, a baked sweet potato delivers a bounty of nutrients with relatively few calories. (Just be sure to avoid adding excessive toppings, such as marshmallows, or you'll pile on empty calories.) Following are some other nutrient-rich foods. You'll notice that these are all unprocessed or minimally processed foods.

- Almonds, cashews, peanuts
- Avocados
- Barley, oats, quinoa, brown rice
- Beans (garbanzo, kidney, navy, pinto)
- Bell peppers
- Berries (blackberries, blueberries, raspberries, strawberries)
- Brussels sprouts
- Cantaloupe, kiwi, papaya
- Chard, collard greens, kale, mustard greens, spinach
- Chicken, turkey
- Eggs
- Lean beef, lamb, venison
- Lentils, peas
- Mushrooms (crimini, shiitake)
- Onions, leeks, garlic
- Salmon, halibut, cod, scallops, tuna
- Seeds (flax, pumpkin, sesame, sunflower)
- Tomatoes
- Yogurt

the Mediterranean diet reduced heart attack, stroke, and death by about 30% compared with a low-fat diet over the course of 4.8 years. Another study examining the relative importance of each component of the Mediterranean diet found that its life-extending benefits stemmed mainly from eating plenty of vegetables, fruits, nuts, legumes, and olive oil; eating little meat; and drinking a glass or two of wine with meals. Another bonus: a two-year-long study found that dieters lost more weight on a Mediterranean diet than a low-fat diet.

Or … try the DASH diet

The DASH (Dietary Approaches to Stop Hypertension) diet was created in the 1990s to help people lower their blood pressure. It has also been shown to help reduce cholesterol levels, and it's been recognized as a healthy eating plan that is easy to follow and adopt.

Like the Mediterranean diet, the DASH diet emphasizes the consumption of vegetables, fruits, fat-free or low-fat dairy products, whole grains, fish, poultry, beans, seeds, nuts, and "good" fats, such as vegetable oils. The dietary plan also recommends reducing the intake of red meats, sodium, sweets, and sugar-containing beverages. For the particulars of the plan, visit www.health.harvard.edu/bp-guide or www.health.harvard.edu/dash.

Make healthful food choices

Some essential nutrients are packed into every food, and certain foods—such as flour, cereal, and salt—are fortified with specific nutrients as well. Vitamin and mineral supplements from a bottle cannot encompass all the biologically active compounds teeming in a well-stocked pantry. A simple apple or floret of broccoli contains scores of nutrients besides vitamins and minerals that might interact to improve your health. For example, broccoli contains compounds called isothiocyanates, which appear to have anti-tumor properties. For more information, see "Phytochemicals (bioactives)," page 36. It also pays to remember the following advice.

Limit liquid sugars

Liquid sugars, which are found in soft drinks, sports drinks, fruit drinks, iced teas, and sweetened waters, have no benefits for health and are clearly linked to a higher risk of obesity, diabetes, and perhaps heart disease. There is no reason to include these in your diet. Skip the sugary drinks—and even artificially sweetened drinks, which also have been associated with deleterious health effects. Have some unsweetened tea or sparkling water instead.

Minimize refined carbohydrates

Highly processed wheat, rice, and other grains have the same effects in the body as table sugar. So minimize your intake of white bread, French fries, most breakfast cereals, and most high-carbohydrate packaged and processed foods, such as pretzels and chips. Instead, choose whole grains, high-fiber breakfast cereals, brown rice, steel-cut oats, and fruits and vegetables. When choosing carbs, a good rule of thumb is to be sure that they have no more than 10 grams of carbohydrate for every gram of dietary fiber (maximum 10-to-1 carbohydrate-to-fiber ratio). Even better,

SPECIAL SECTION | Does your diet deliver the daily recommended dose?

> ### Getting the most from foods
>
> Whether you're a gourmet chef or a novice in the kitchen, you can learn to squeeze the most nutritional benefit from your diet. Choosing nutritious foods is the most important step, but the following tips can help you preserve the nutritional content of your foods:
>
> **Don't forgo frozen or canned.** The fruits and vegetables stocked in supermarket freezer aisles are usually picked ripe and flash frozen, which captures their flavor and seals in nutrients. And larger stores carry everything from old standards like frozen blueberries or chopped broccoli to newer additions like frozen turnip greens, gooseberries, and plantains. Canned fruits and vegetables are also a good alternative, but make sure to choose products that are canned in water and low in salt and sugar.
>
> **Steam, stir-fry, grill, or roast vegetables.** Boiling veggies can lead to a loss of nutrients into the cooking water. But don't get caught up in little details of the "best" way to prepare vegetables. The key step is to buy them and eat them—you'll be doing your body a favor no matter how you prepare them.
>
> **Wrap it up.** Properly store or refrigerate any cut fruits or vegetables in order to ensure that they will last and retain their key nutrients. Cap juice bottles.
>
> **Cook it well.** Foods such as meat, fish, and poultry must be cooked well in order to destroy dangerous microorganisms. If you grill your food, be sure not to char it, in order to avoid formation of cancer-causing compounds.

if possible, aim for no more than 5 grams of carbohydrate for every gram of dietary fiber (maximum 5-to-1 carbohydrate-to-fiber ratio).

Choose healthy fats

Fish, nuts, and vegetable oils contain healthy monounsaturated and polyunsaturated fats, which help lower heart disease risk. Eat these foods regularly and in moderation. Don't focus on the amount of fat (for example, low-fat salad dressing), but rather the type of fat. Limit your consumption of saturated fat and cholesterol, and especially avoid eating trans fat, found in partially hydrogenated vegetable oils (used in spreads, baked goods, and fast foods). Trans fats are being phased out of the U.S. food supply, but will still be in some products on store shelves until Jan. 1, 2020.

Don't forget fiber

Eat plenty of foods that contain dietary fiber (the edible, indigestible parts of plant foods). Good sources include fruits, vegetables, whole grains, beans, and nuts. Fiber from grains helps lower the risk of heart disease. Your daily fiber goal depends on your age and sex, as follows:

- men ages 50 or younger: 38 grams
- men over 50: 30 grams
- women ages 50 or younger: 25 grams
- women over 50: 21 grams.

Balance energy intake and output

To keep your weight stable, the energy you take in should equal the energy you use. That means if you are sedentary, you need far fewer calories to remain at your current weight than someone the same height and weight who is active.

Favor fruits and vegetables

Most Americans don't eat nearly the recommended amounts of fruits and vegetables (see Figure 5, page 43). Preparation time, unfamiliarity, and old habits are common hurdles. Here are some suggestions to break these barriers and boost your intake.

Set a goal. Start by eating one extra fruit or vegetable a day. When you're used to that, add another and keep going. For example, add fruit to your breakfast cereal every morning. Then try eating a piece of fruit for an after-lunch snack. Next, add at least one vegetable to your dinner plate.

Be sneaky. Adding finely grated carrots or zucchini to pasta sauce, meat loaf, chili, or a stew is one way to get an extra serving of vegetables.

Try something new. It's easy to get tired of apples, bananas, and grapes. Try a kiwi, mango, fresh pineapple, or some of the more exotic choices now found in many grocery stores. The same goes for vegetables. You might find you love kale, leeks, or bok choy.

Blend in. A fruit smoothie (see "Simple fruit smoothie," page 41) is a delicious way to start the day or tide you over until dinner. You can add spinach to a fruit smoothie without sacrificing the sweet taste.

Be a big dipper. Try dipping vegetables into hummus or another

Does your diet deliver the daily recommended dose? | **SPECIAL SECTION**

bean spread, some spiced yogurt, or even a bit of ranch dressing. Slather peanut butter on a banana or slices of apple. Dip fresh or dried fruit in melted dark chocolate.

Spread it on. Try mashed avocado as a dip with diced tomatoes and onions, or as a sandwich spread, topped with spinach leaves, tomatoes, and a slice of cheese.

Start off right. Ditch your morning donut for an omelet with onions, peppers, and mushrooms. Top it with some salsa to wake up your palate. Or boost your morning cereal or oatmeal with a handful of strawberries, blueberries, or dried fruit.

Drink up. Having a 6-ounce glass of low-sodium vegetable juice instead of a soda gives you a full serving of vegetables and spares you 10 teaspoons or more of sugar. You can also make your own vegetable juice with a blender or juicer.

Give them the heat treatment. Roasting vegetables is easy and brings out new flavors. Cut up onions, carrots, zucchini, asparagus, turnips—whatever you have on hand—coat with olive oil, add a dash of balsamic vinegar, and roast at 350° until done. Grilling is another way to bring out the taste of vegetables. Use roasted or grilled vegetables as a side dish, put them on sandwiches, or add them to salads.

Let someone else do the work. If peeling, cutting, and chopping are too time-consuming, food companies and grocers offer an ever-expanding selection of prepared produce, from ready-made salads to frozen stir-fry mixes and take-along sliced apples and dip.

Improve on nature. Don't hesitate to jazz up vegetables with spices, chopped nuts, balsamic vinegar, olive oil, or a specialty oil like walnut or sesame oil. Most grocers carry several spice blends made specifically for vegetables. Even a dash of grated Parmesan cheese can liven up the blandest green beans.

Decoding your diet

If you're really curious to know how your diet stacks up nutrition-wise, you have two options: hire a professional or do it yourself.

A registered dietitian can scrutinize your current diet and set up a plan that precisely meets your nutritional needs, taking into consideration your food preferences and allergies or other health issues (such as lactose intolerance or celiac disease). Many dietitians have access to computer programs and databases that ease the most difficult calculations, such as nutrient analyses of menus. You can ask your clinician for a referral (check to see if your insurance covers the cost of nutritional counseling), or ask at a local hospital or medical center.

But if you have the time and the inclination to do the work yourself, there are free online tools and calculators that can help. Here are some questions you'll need to ask and some of the websites where you can find the answers.

Simple fruit smoothie

Makes: 1 serving

This is a great way to use bananas that are beginning to get too ripe. (You can always cut ripe bananas into thick slices, freeze in a plastic bag, and thaw when you're ready to make another smoothie.)

- ¾ cup plain yogurt or kefir
- ½ cup berries (fresh or frozen strawberries, blueberries, or other berry of your choice)
- ½ ripe banana
- ½ cup pineapple juice

Optional: 1 tablespoon ground flaxseed (for healthy omega-3 fats).

Put all ingredients in a blender or food processor and blend to combine. You can branch out by adding a dash of ground cinnamon, a splash of vanilla, some mint, or another flavoring.

How many calories do I need?

It depends on your age, height, weight, and activity level. You can get a rough estimate of how many calories you need each day to maintain your weight by simply multiplying your weight by a value ranging from 11 to 15, depending on whether you are short or tall, sedentary or active, and so forth. For a more precise figure, try the calculator at Calculator.net (www.calculator.net/calorie-calculator.html).

What should I eat?

For a list of nutrient-dense foods you can incorporate into your diet, go to the World's Healthiest Foods (www.whfoods.com/foodstoc.php). Another good source of informa-

Continued on page 43

SPECIAL SECTION | Does your diet deliver the daily recommended dose?

A typical diet vs. a nutrient-dense diet

If you want to meet your vitamin and mineral requirements through diet rather than supplements—by far the best way to do it—your best bet is to adopt a nutrient-dense diet. But for someone who hasn't already been eating this way, it might not be obvious how to do that. The two menus below show how one 52-year-old woman managed the shift, with the help of clinical dietitian Ellen di Bonaventura at Harvard-affiliated Massachusetts General Hospital in Boston.

The "typical day's menu" shows the kind of regimen the woman was following before consulting di Bonaventura. The "nutrient-dense menu" shows a typical day's diet after she overhauled her eating to include more produce. Note that she boosted her nutrients into the recommended range without relying on fortified food products or supplements. At the same time, she slashed calories from roughly 2,000 a day to just under 1,200—a level often recommended for female dieters.

A typical day's menu

Breakfast
1 whole-wheat bagel
2 tablespoons light cream cheese
10 ounces coffee
2 ounces skim milk
6 ounces nonfat strawberry yogurt

Lunch
2 slices oatmeal bread
1 tablespoon light mayonnaise
4 ounces tuna, canned in water
1 ounce chips
12 ounces diet cola

Snack
1 oat-and-honey granola bar
6 ounces black tea with 1 teaspoon milk and ½ teaspoon sugar

Menu provides 1,959 calories:
32% from fat
43% from carbohydrate
20% from protein
5% from alcohol

Dinner
5 ounces grilled chicken marinated in 2 tablespoons Italian dressing
½ cup white rice
1 tablespoon margarine
1 cup broccoli florets
5 ounces white wine

Dessert
½ ounce dark chocolate

Nutrient analysis of this menu

The amounts of vitamins and minerals this woman consumed through her diet are shown below, next to the recommended daily amounts in parentheses. Shortfalls are noted in bold.

Vitamin A, 529 mcg (700 mcg)	Vitamin K, 137 mcg (90 mcg)
Thiamin, 1.5 mg (1.1 mg)	**Calcium, 477 mg (1,200 mg)**
Riboflavin, 1.8 mg (1.1 mg)	**Copper, 881 mcg (900 mcg)**
Niacin, 52 mg (14 mg)	Iron, 13 mg (8 mg)
Pantothenic acid, 4.6 mg (5 mg)	**Magnesium, 268 mg (320 mg)**
Vitamin B_6, 1.3 mg (1.5 mg)	Manganese, 5.1 mg (1.8 mg)
Folate, 379 mcg (400 mcg)	Phosphorus, 1,148 mg (700 mg)
Vitamin B_{12}, 4.0 mcg (2.4 mcg)	**Potassium, 2,000 mg (4,700 mg)**
Vitamin C, 44 mg (75 mg)	Selenium, 179 mcg (55 mcg)
Vitamin D, 280 IU (600 IU)	**Zinc, 7.2 mg (8 mg)**

A nutrient-dense menu

Breakfast
8 ounces nonfat yogurt
½ cup sliced papaya
½ cup sliced kiwi
1 ounce (14 halves) walnuts
8 ounces black coffee
4 ounces skim milk

Lunch
1 small whole-wheat pita
Green salad (1 cup dark green lettuce, 1 red or orange pepper, 1 cup grape tomatoes, ½ cup edamame beans, 1 tablespoon unsalted sunflower seeds)
Salad dressing (1 tablespoon olive oil plus balsamic vinegar and pepper)
Unsweetened iced tea or water

Menu provides 1,155 calories:
33% from fat
40% from carbohydrate
27% from protein

Dinner
4 ounces broiled wild salmon and yogurt sauce (1 tablespoon Greek nonfat yogurt, 1 teaspoon lemon juice, 1 clove chopped garlic)
¼ cup cooked barley
¼ cup cooked lentils with spices to taste
1 cup steamed baby bok choy
Water

Nutrient analysis of this menu

The amounts of vitamins and minerals this woman consumed through her new diet are shown below, next to the recommended daily amounts in parentheses. Note that there is now only one nutrient shortfall—vitamin D, which can be hard to obtain through food.

You may not want such a calorie-restricted diet. For example, you might want to add healthy snacks of fruit or a handful of nuts. The point is that you can reduce your calories while boosting nutrient intakes.

Vitamin A, 1,031 mcg (700 mcg)	Vitamin K, 156 mcg (90 mcg)
Thiamin, 1.3 mg (1.1 mg)	Calcium, 1,222 mg (1,200 mg)
Riboflavin, 1.8 mg (1.1 mg)	Copper, 900 mcg (900 mcg)
Niacin, 14 mg (14 mg)	Iron, 11 mg (8 mg)
Pantothenic acid, 5.5 mg (5 mg)	Magnesium, 355 mg (320 mg)
Vitamin B_6, 2.23 mg (1.5 mg)	Manganese, 2.8 mg (1.8 mg)
Folate, 556 mcg (400 mcg)	Phosphorus, 1,530 mg (700 mg)
Vitamin B_{12}, 10.6 mcg (2.4 mcg)	Potassium, 4,700 mg (4,700 mg)
Vitamin C, 383 mg (75 mg)	Selenium, 90 mcg (55 mcg)
Vitamin D, 480 IU (600 IU)	Zinc, 8.6 mg (8 mg)

Does your diet deliver the daily recommended dose? | **SPECIAL SECTION**

Continued from page 41

tion on the nutrients in specific foods (including brand-name and fast-food items) is Calorie King (www.calorieking.com).

How do I know if my diet provides what I need?

To look up the nutrient content of specific foods—or to find out which foods contain specific nutrients—go to the USDA National Nutrient Database for Standard Reference at http://ndb.nal.usda.gov. You can also research the nutrient content of various foods using the Nutrition Facts section of the consumer website for Blue Cross and Blue Shield of Massachusetts (www.ahealthyme.com/Library/NutritionFacts). Entering everything you eat can be cumbersome, but if you try it for just a few days, you'll learn a lot about food quality and how to get the best nutritional return on the calories you consume.

Alternatively, you can take a more relaxed approach—not worrying too much about the details and focusing instead on the big picture: eating a balanced diet that is packed with nutrient-dense foods.

Putting it into practice

Sometimes it seems that you can't possibly meet all your daily requirements for vitamins and minerals from food without vastly increasing the amount of food (and calories) you consume. Rest assured, you can. The single most important step you can take to meet your goal is simply to increase your intake of fruits and vegetables. If you look at "A typical diet vs. a nutrient-dense diet" on page 42, you'll see how one dietitian managed to make over the diet of a 52-year-old woman, boosting her nutrient intake while actually reducing the woman's daily calorie intake.

Notice that this woman was initially consuming the recommended daily amounts for only about half the vitamins and minerals (nine out of 20). That's because her diet included less than half of the recommended servings of vegetables and no fruit at all. But once she switched to the nutrient-dense diet, which is rich in vegetables, fruits, and lean protein, she began meeting all but one of her nutrient goals, including 1,200 mg of calcium a day, thanks to foods such as non-fat dairy products and bok choy (Chinese cabbage). ♥

Figure 5: A diet out of balance

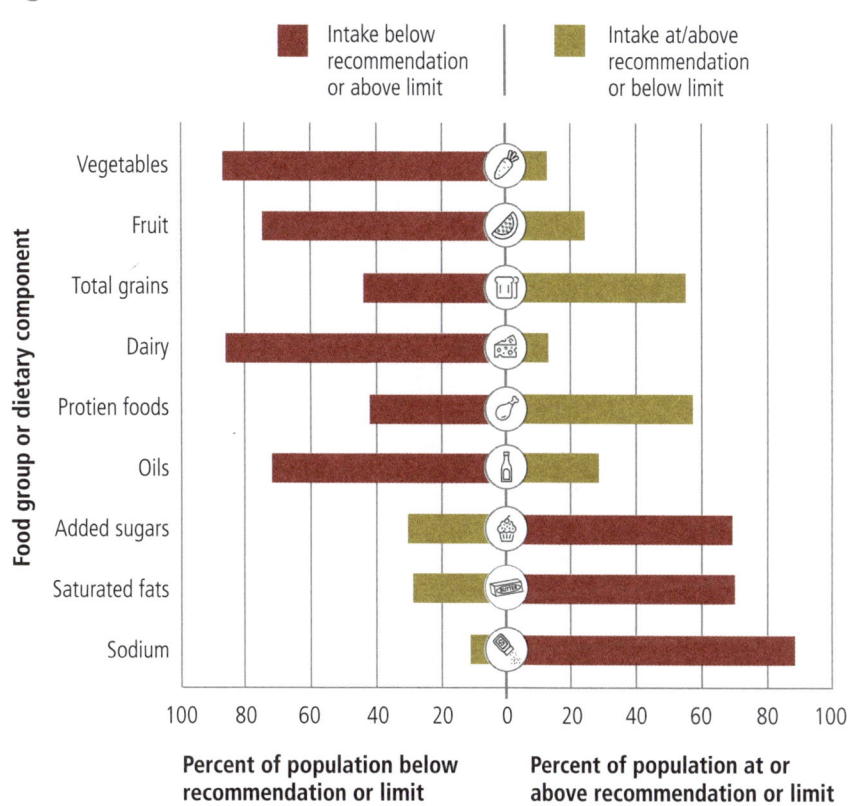

In general, Americans tend to eat more nutrient-poor foods, like sweetened drinks and other sweets, and not enough foods that are rich in vitamins, minerals, and other nutrients.

Source: Dietary Guidelines for Americans, 2015–2020.

www.health.harvard.edu

Making Sense of Vitamins and Minerals 43

Getting too little

Serious deficiencies of most essential vitamins and minerals are relatively rare in America, although they do occur in some pockets of the country. More often, people get enough to avoid overt deficiency ailments such as scurvy or rickets, but because of nutrient-poor diets, they get too little of some nutrients to help ward off chronic health problems, such as osteoporosis, cardiovascular disease, and some types of cancer. How can you tell if you could be compromising your health by not getting enough? While definitive proof is hard to come by, there are certain clues.

Age

According to the Framingham Heart Study, 30% of people ages 67 and over lack adequate folic acid, 20% do not get sufficient vitamin B_6, and 20% to 25% do not get enough B_{12}. The Baltimore Longitudinal Study on Aging found that most older men and women are deficient in calcium, zinc, iron, magnesium, and vitamin D. Malabsorption, poor diet, or other causes may underpin this pervasive problem. A lack of stomach acid—which often occurs among the elderly—makes it hard to absorb calcium and vitamin B_{12} from food.

Sex

Women who menstruate need more iron compared with men, postmenopausal women, and women who've had a hysterectomy. Because most of the body's iron circulates in the blood as part of hemoglobin, menstruating girls and women lose substantial amounts of iron during their monthly periods, which is why iron deficiency is a common problem for women of childbearing age. For women ages 31 to 50, the recommended daily amount of iron is 18 mg. For adult men of any age and for women starting at age 50 (or whenever menstruation ends), 8 mg a day is enough.

Any woman who might get pregnant also needs extra folic acid. During the first three weeks of pregnancy, folic acid is essential in preventing birth defects of the brain and spine. Some research suggests that the daily dose for women of childbearing age should be 800 mcg, not the 400 mcg currently recommended and present in most multivitamins. Combining a healthy diet with a multivitamin should provide you with about 700 to 800 mcg a day.

Medical conditions

Some digestive diseases can block absorption of vitamin B_{12}. Cystic fibrosis, chronic liver disease, and short-bowel syndrome can impair the absorption of fat-soluble vitamins, such as vitamin E. Liver disease, kidney disease, or malabsorption maladies can trigger a deficiency of vitamin K, which is essential for blood clotting and may help keep bones healthy. Celiac disease, inflammatory bowel disease, and other conditions that affect the small intestine can interfere with vitamin D absorption. In addition, medications can interfere with the absorption of some vitamins and minerals (see "Medications and micronutrients," page 45).

Genes

People lacking a particular gene variant—which leads to having a less-active form of an enzyme that helps the body use folic acid—have a higher risk for colorectal cancer when they take in too little of this B vitamin. Other genetic abnormalities hamper the body's ability to make and use vitamin D, thus increasing the risk for bone fractures.

Vegetarian and vegan diets

Unlike every other vitamin, B_{12} is almost exclusively found in animal products (eggs, milk, fish, poultry, and meat). Vegans and strict vegetarians court a B_{12} deficiency, which can inflict neurological damage and contribute to heart disease. Taking a multivitamin will solve the problem. Vegetarians who aren't quite so strict—who avoid meat, but eat milk and eggs—can get their B_{12} that way. People who follow a plant-based diet should also eat plenty of deep-hued vegetables and fruits, to ensure that they get enough essential vitamins and minerals, along with other healthful compounds.

Alcohol consumption

Heavy drinking is known to cause folic acid deficiency. It can also contribute to deficiencies of vitamin A, thiamin, vitamin D, magnesium, calcium, and potassium. And tissue studies show it may increase the need for niacin, vitamin C, and sometimes zinc.

Even moderate drinking—no more than one drink per day for women and two for men—may pose a problem. Women in the Nurses' Health Study who drank moderate amounts of alcohol and took in little folic acid had a higher risk for breast cancer than their counterparts who took multivitamins containing folic acid. This combination—drinking alcohol and having low levels of folic acid—has been linked to colon cancer, too. Experts advise even moderate consumers of alcohol to step up their folic acid intake, for example by taking a regular multivitamin that contains folate.

There is a complex pattern of risks and benefits associated with alcohol use, and because alcohol lacks vitamins and minerals, drinking doesn't translate into an overall healthy food choice. And although the media has brought attention to the potential health benefits of the bioactive compounds in red wine and other alcoholic beverages, the promise is far greater than the actual findings from research conducted to date.

A systematic analysis of the worldwide burden of alcohol use published in 2018 in *The Lancet* provides additional evidence that alcohol should be kept to a minimum: it found that alcohol use may increase the risk of various cancers and overall mortality, and this risk increases as consumption rises. The only level of alcohol consumption that was associated with zero health risks was zero consumption.

The bottom line on alcohol is to stick to the current guidelines of no more than one drink per day for women and two drinks per day for men—and not to start drinking if you don't currently consume alcohol.

Blood loss

When you lose blood, you lose iron, too. Women who menstruate need extra iron. So do frequent blood donors—an estimated 3 to 4 mg more per day for each unit of blood you donate during the course of a year. Talk with your doctor if you donate regularly.

Medications and micronutrients

Some medications can interfere with the absorption of certain nutrients or speed their excretion from the body. You're more likely to suffer from nutrient depletion and worrisome interactions if you take several medications, regularly drink alcohol, eat poorly, or have health problems that increase your need for certain nutrients.

It's also true that certain nutrients in food and supplements can interfere with the medications you take. Prime examples are calcium and iron, which bind to the antibiotic tetracycline so that both the nutrients and the drug simply pass through the body in an unusable form. Megadoses of vitamin C can acidify your urine, which curbs the excretion of acidic drugs, such as aspirin. That means the aspirin will stay in your body longer than usual.

Generally, when you begin using a medication, your pharmacist should warn you about any foods to avoid. But you should never take a dietary supplement without finding out whether it might interfere or interact with the medications you take. Ask your pharmacist or doctor—not the clerk at a health-food store—for this information. It helps to buy all your prescription drugs and supplements at one pharmacy, especially if the store maintains computerized customer records to track possible drug interactions.

The following classes of medications may cause nutrient depletion and, possibly, nutritional deficiencies. (If you take any of these medicines, ask your doctor whether you should adjust your intake of any vitamins or minerals. Generally, occasional use will not matter, but long-term use can make a difference.)

- antacids
- antibacterial agents
- antibiotics
- anticancer drugs
- anticoagulants
- anticonvulsants
- antidepressants
- antifungal agents
- anti-inflammatory agents
- antimalarials
- anti-ulcer drugs
- cholesterol-lowering medications
- contraceptives
- corticosteroids
- diabetes medications
- diuretics
- laxatives
- tranquilizers.

Getting too much

While getting too little of essential micronutrients can harm your health over the long haul, getting too much can have equally worrisome effects, many of which show up more swiftly. Most troublesome are excesses of fat-soluble vitamins from supplements, which the body may stockpile to the point of toxicity. The ones most likely to cause trouble are vitamins A, E, and K. (D is also fat-soluble, but an excess of D doesn't tend to cause problems.)

High doses of supplements—usually from taking individual vitamin and mineral supplements in addition to a powerful multivitamin—are often at fault. It's much harder to get dangerous amounts of micronutrients from food, partly because of the body's natural checks and balances. When iron stores are full, for example, your body absorbs less iron from food unless a genetic disorder or other problem interferes. Your body also slows the conversion of beta carotene to vitamin A when it already has enough vitamin A from supplements or food sources. But it is still possible to overdo it.

Many consumers are spurred to take excessive supplement doses by overenthusiastic news stories on the potential benefits of certain vitamins and minerals. Remember, though, that the good news from the latest study may be refuted by other studies. Promising test-tube and animal studies often don't pan out in people. And certain types of human studies offer more definitive information than others. Sometimes, exciting results from initial observational studies aren't confirmed by randomized controlled trials, which are considered the gold standard of research. And even these studies often have their limitations.

The bottom line is clear: Don't take more than the recommended dose of any micronutrient through supplements unless there is a good reason to do so, such as specific advice from your doctor, dietitian, or other qualified health professional. It is especially important to avoid taking too much of the following vitamins and minerals.

Vitamin A

It can be easy to ingest 10,000 IU (3,000 mcg) of vitamin A—more than three times the amount recommended for men and four times the amount recommended for women—if you eat a lot of fortified cereal and liver in addition to taking a multivitamin containing retinol or retinyl compounds every day.

Plenty of evidence from earlier research shows that too much vitamin A can harm bones. Excess vitamin A can have other effects as well. Birth defects occur more often when pregnant women take more than 10,000 IU of supplemental vitamin A. To protect yourself, get most or all of your supplemental vitamin A in the form of beta carotene, and try to stick to the RDA for vitamin A.

Vitamin E

Despite evidence that vitamin E supplements don't help and may even be harmful (see "Vitamin E," page 26), some people still take these supplements. If you take more than 1,200 IU (800 mg) per day, you risk side

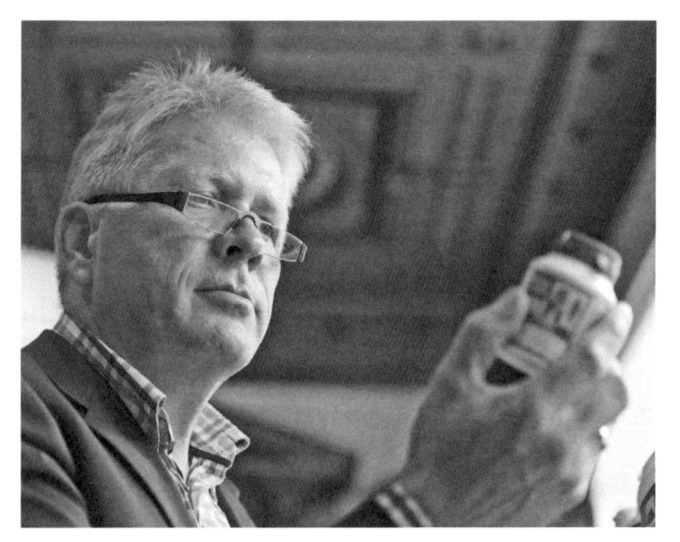

When you rely on supplements rather than food to meet your nutrient requirements, it can be easy to take too much.

effects such as bleeding, headache, fatigue, and blurred vision. To be on the safe side, talk with your doctor before taking more than the RDA for vitamin E to avoid increasing your risk of bleeding, especially if you also take the blood thinner warfarin (Coumadin).

Vitamin K

Because vitamin K can influence blood clotting, if you take warfarin it's important to keep your vitamin K intake consistent from day to day. Discuss this with your doctor if you are taking this medication.

Calcium (for men)

There is some evidence that a high intake of calcium may increase the risk of prostate cancer and may also increase heart attack risk, though no randomized trials have specifically tested the latter. One study found that men who consumed more than 2,000 mg of calcium daily were five times as likely to develop metastatic prostate cancer as those who consumed less than 500 mg of calcium per day. Another large epidemiological study found that intake of more than 1,500 mg of calcium per day might increase the risk of aggressive and fatal prostate cancer, but not the risk of less aggressive, localized cancer. As there are many food sources of calcium available, men should avoid taking calcium supplements unless there are concerns about insufficient intake—which would warrant a discussion with your physician or a nutritionist.

Iron

Hemochromatosis is the medical term for too much iron in the body. A common genetic glitch called hereditary hemochromatosis leaves about 1.5 million Americans prone to a glut of iron, although not automatically doomed to it. Large doses of iron supplements, multiple blood transfusions, drinking too much alcohol, and some rare metabolic disorders can also trigger an iron overload, which can damage body tissues and raise risks for infection, heart disease, liver cancer, and arthritis over time.

In addition, taking high doses of vitamin C allows your body to absorb more iron than it normally would accept and release more stored iron than necessary. This causes an upswing in free iron, which attacks DNA, cell lipids, and protein. Free iron also results when abnormally high levels of iron accumulate in the body for other reasons.

Excess iron is not easily shed. More men than women suffer from an overabundance of iron; in fact, men are twice as likely to have iron overload than iron deficiency.

The tolerable upper intake level for iron is 45 mg a day. A child who takes as few as five pills each containing 200 mg of iron can die from poisoning. Any supplements that contain iron—especially chewable children's multivitamins that look like candy—should be stored well away from children.

Zinc

Getting enough—but not too much—of the trace mineral zinc is a bit of a high-wire act. The RDA for zinc is 8 mg for women and 11 mg for men. The Health and Medicine Division of the National Academies of Sciences, Engineering, and Medicine lists the upper limit for zinc as 40 mg for women and men. Yet levels not much higher than 15 mg can trigger side effects, such as a depressed immune system, poor healing, hair loss, and interference with the ability to taste and smell. That's why some experts suggest that it's best to get zinc from food sources rather than supplements. At the very least, make sure that your multivitamin provides no more than 15 mg of zinc. And be sure to count zinc intake from lozenges if you take them during a cold, which can easily put you over the upper limit for this mineral.

Your overall diet affects how much zinc your body typically absorbs from food. Interestingly, you are likely to absorb less zinc if you choose a diet rich in healthy whole grains and with very little animal protein. Most North Americans probably absorb about 38% of available dietary zinc.

So, should you take supplements?

In the 1980s, many nutritionists and some physicians began to recommend (and take) vitamin supplements. However, as described earlier in this report, the evidence for the health benefits of most supplements is not strong. And taking individual supplements, in general, is not advised unless your health care provider or a dietitian recommends it. Notable exceptions are vitamin D for bone health and folic acid during pregnancy. Although foods that contain vitamin A and beta carotene, as well as vitamins B, C, and E, are clearly good for health, taking supplements of these vitamins has no proven health benefits.

What about a simple multivitamin-multimineral supplement—a product that is designed to meet the RDAs and to compensate for dietary shortfalls? "Multis" are the most popular among all dietary supplements—half of Americans take them on a regular basis, shelling out more than $20 billion annually on these products. On an individual basis, a daily multivitamin won't set you back that much: a year's supply of many popular brands costs about $30 to $50.

However, the composition of these tablets varies widely, with some containing all of the essential vitamins and minerals, and some containing just a few of them. And despite the widespread belief that multivitamin-multimineral supplements will prevent chronic diseases such as cancer and heart disease, the U.S. Preventive Services Task Force has concluded that there isn't enough evidence to support such claims.

The main reason for this conclusion is that only one large-scale, long-term randomized controlled trial—the Physicians' Health Study II of male doctors—tested the effects of a regular multivitamin. In that trial, regardless of the quality of their diets, men who took a daily multi for over a decade had *no less* risk of having a heart attack or stroke or dying of cardiovascular disease than those who did not take one. However, they did have an 8% reduction in cancer and a 9% reduction in the development of cataracts.

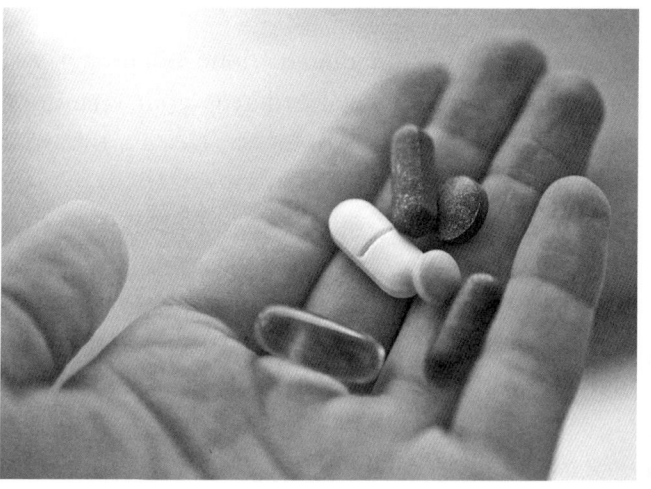

The FDA does not certify supplements for safety or effectiveness as it does for drugs, nor does it set potency or dosage standards. Manufacturers are left to police themselves.

If there is one place you would expect a benefit to show up, it would be in observational studies, but these, too, show no benefit to taking multis. For example, in the Nurses' Health Study—a prospective, 32-year observational trial of 86,142 women—the use of multis was not found to reduce the incidence of stroke or death, even in women with a poor-quality diet—the very women who should gain the most from taking supplements. And a recent meta-analysis published in the *Journal of the American College of Cardiology* reported that there was limited evidence on multivitamin-multimineral supplements for preventing or treating cardiovascular disease.

The upshot of this is that we need more high-quality, large-scale research to evaluate the benefits of multivitamin-multimineral supplements—and a new large randomized trial called the Cocoa Supplement and Multivitamin Outcomes Study (COSMOS) is now under way to do that. Researchers at Harvard University and the Fred Hutchinson Cancer Center in Seattle have recruited 21,444 women ages 65 and older and men 60 and older, and are testing a commonly used multivitamin-multimineral supplement and a cocoa extract supplement in a trial that is anticipated to last four years.

The good news is that of all vitamin or mineral supplements you could take, a standard multivitamin-multimineral supplement has the fewest potential downsides and the most potential benefits for your health. In addition, taking one is already part of some official recommendations. The federal government's Dietary Guidelines for Americans suggest that people over age 50 consider a vitamin B_{12} supplement or a multi as a way to ensure adequate vitamin B_{12} intake. And the Centers for Disease Control and Prevention advises all women of childbearing age to take folic acid—typically included in a multi—because doing so lowers the risk of birth defects (see "Folic acid," page 19).

When choosing a multi, look for an inexpensive preparation from a mainstream manufacturer to ensure quality and consistency. It should contain 100% of the DV for vitamin D, vitamin B_6, vitamin B_{12}, and folic acid. Extra vitamin D is unlikely to be harmful—as noted earlier, many experts recommend 1,000 IU, which is almost twice the DV, and is now found in many formulations. But extra amounts of other vitamins may do more harm than good.

What about supplements aimed at women, men, and seniors? While some of these formulas may be helpful in certain cases, others are merely marketing gimmicks designed to enhance profits rather than your health. Products vary widely; read the labels to make sure you get what you need while staying within safe limits for your age and sex.

Don't waste your money on high-potency, "all natural," or designer vitamins. Above all, remember that your daily multi is at least an insurance policy—a supplement, not a substitute, for a healthful diet—that may or may not provide long-term health benefits.

Potential pitfalls of supplement use

Shopping for any kind of supplement can be confusing. A staggering array of multivitamins and other supplements crowd the shelves of pharmacies, grocery stores, and specialty stores, and many more are now available over the Internet. Before you buy, it's wise to realize that some of these products may offer much more—or possibly less—than you really need to enhance your health.

Dietary supplements may legally contain vitamins, minerals, herbs, amino acids, enzymes, organ

Understanding health claims on labels

Many foods, beverages, vitamin and mineral supplements, and other products tout impressive claims about their potential health benefits. Unlike prescription medications, which must go through a series of safety and efficacy trials before receiving FDA approval, foods and supplements do not routinely undergo the same level of scrutiny. Here are the four types of health claims they tout—and what they actually mean.

Nutrient content claims describe the amount of a specific nutrient in a food product—for example, free of saturated fat, high in vitamin C, or low in sugar. However, just because a food is low in saturated fat, that does not stop it from having high levels of sugar, for example.

Structure and function claims describe how dietary components of a food product may affect structures or functions of the body. They tend to be general in nature. For instance, a food with antioxidants may maintain cell integrity, but how does that translate to your overall health?

Qualified health claims describe how particular foods or nutrients affect specific health outcomes and offer greater supportive evidence than structure and function claims. A food or supplement manufacturer must submit a petition to the FDA with sufficient research to support the approval of that qualified health claim. While a qualified health claim must be supported by *some* scientific evidence, it does not necessarily meet the higher standard for *significant* scientific agreement. As a result, qualified health claims must be accompanied by a disclaimer—for example, "Whole grains may reduce the risk of type 2 diabetes, although the FDA has concluded that there is very limited scientific evidence for this claim."

Authorized health claims are a step above qualified health claims and must have *significant* scientific agreement among qualified experts, with publicly available scientific evidence submitted to the FDA to back them up. These claims describe a relationship between a specific food, food component, or nutrient with a disease or health-related condition. For example, "Diets low in sodium may reduce the risk of high blood pressure, a disease associated with many factors."

tissues, and a few other substances—in short, practically any ingredient promoted as a way to bolster your diet and, presumably, your health. The FDA does not certify supplements for safety or effectiveness in the same way it monitors drugs. Under the Dietary Supplement Health and Education Act of 1994, the FDA does not have the authority to approve supplements or demand that manufacturers undertake rigorous studies to prove their worth. The FDA doesn't set potency or dosage standards, either.

Manufacturers are left to police themselves. And before a worrisome supplement can be pulled off the market, the FDA has to prove that it creates a significant health risk. This can lead to problems, as is made clear by a report from ConsumerLab.com, an industry watchdog organization. The organization tested the quality and contents of 75 leading multivitamin and multimineral products for adults and children sold in the United States and Canada. Almost half of the products did not receive the group's approval. Gummies had the lowest quality of all products tested, often containing far more or far less of listed nutrients than the label claimed. (Some variation in the amount of vitamins and minerals in a product is to be expected because supplements will slowly and naturally degrade over the course of their shelf life; pay attention to expiration dates on the packaging.) Moreover, some tablet products did not disintegrate quickly enough for all nutrients to be absorbed in the gut.

While supplement manufacturers can't legally claim to prevent, treat, or cure specific diseases, they can come pretty close. They are allowed to make "structure-function" claims that sound impressive to most consumers. A product may "build strong teeth" or "improve memory" or "boost the immune system." Manufacturers can make these assertions without supplying a stitch of proof to any agency. Your cue for healthy skepticism should be the words printed alongside: "This statement has not been evaluated by the Food and Drug Administration."

Certain health claims backed by substantial scientific agreement and not limited to particular brands can appear on supplement bottles. For example, supplement manufacturers can advertise that "calcium helps protect against osteoporosis" and "folic acid may prevent neural tube defects in fetuses," because these statements are borne out by science and have been carefully evaluated (see "Understanding health claims on labels," page 49).

Advice on choosing a supplement

Buying supplements can raise many questions. Should you choose supplements derived from natural ingredients? Do brand-name supplements have any advantage over less expensive store brands? Are the health claims plausible? Are the suggested dosages safe? The following advice should help answer these questions and guide you as you make your choices.

Consider your particular nutrient needs. Then do a little sleuthing. Start by checking the label of your multivitamin-multimineral supplement, looking at the recommended amounts listed in Tables 1 and 2 (starting on page 9), and assessing your diet (see "Decoding your diet," page 41). Are you getting too little vitamin D? Need extra calcium? Looking for lutein or other potentially beneficial phytochemicals? Your first line of defense should be through food. Rearrange your diet to include more sources of the nutrients you're lacking. For those nutrients that may be hard to get through food, such as vitamin D and calcium, consider buying separate supplements.

Look for a seal of approval. Choose products that bear the U.S. Pharmacopeia Dietary Supplement Verification Program (USP-DSVP) mark, which indicates that the supplement manufacturer has complied with certain standards. Supplements vetted by the USP-DSVP should contain the ingredients noted on the label in the amounts and strengths stated. The product should dissolve within 30 to 45 minutes so that the nutrients enter your bloodstream, rather than passing through your body intact. It shouldn't contain more than allowable levels of contaminants. Other product safety organizations include ConsumerLab.com, which ranks herbs and

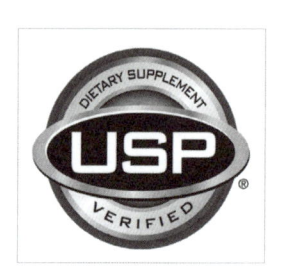

The U.S. Pharmacopeia Dietary Supplement Verification Program (USP-DSVP) mark

supplements based on quality and content, and NSF International, a nonprofit organization that develops standards and certifies products related to public health, safety, and environmental protection.

Consider safe levels. Supplements vary so widely, it's essential to read the labels. Much like packaged foods, which have a Nutrition Facts label, all dietary supplements have a Supplement Facts label that lists the DVs of nutrients in a single serving. It also notes the actual amount of each nutrient included. For trace minerals, such as iron, fluoride, and zinc, it's safest not to exceed the DV at all. Some experts even recommend getting these micronutrients only through food. If you take individual supplements (such as extra vitamin D tablets) as well as a multivitamin, be sure to total up the amounts you're getting from every source, including food. Fortified breakfast cereals can bump up your intake of vitamins and minerals considerably. A single serving of certain breakfast cereals can deliver as much as or more than your daily multivitamin. That may not be a problem with vitamin C, but it might pose health risks with iron or vitamin A.

Consider price. Compare active ingredients on the labels, then let price be your guide. Store brands spend less on advertising than nationally known brands and pass on the savings to the consumer.

Ignore marketing gimmicks. It doesn't matter whether vitamin C is derived from organic rose hips or synthesized in large batches in a laboratory; your body will use the resulting product similarly. In fact, your body absorbs certain micronutrients more efficiently in synthetic rather than natural forms. Vitamin K and folic acid are two examples. If you're not sensitive to specific ingredients, such as wheat, rice, or lactose, there's no need to pay more for allergen-free products. "High potency" isn't a plus in cases when more is not better.

Keep it simple! If you feel compelled to take a handful of supplements each day, consider the bigger picture of how to improve or fine-tune your overall diet. Meet with a nutritionist or start with your primary care provider for guidance.

Avoid gummy vitamins, unless you cannot swallow pills. Gummies typically contain fewer vitamins and minerals and in lower amounts than multivitamin tablets. Plus you have to take them twice a day, they have more calories and added sugar, and they are not as cost-effective as tablets, since a single gummy costs more than a supplement pill.

Don't pay more for unproven extras. Generally, if you're hoping for phytochemical benefits, you'll do better in the produce department than the supplement aisle. There is virtually no evidence that herbs and other nonvitamin ingredients added to supplements are essential for your health. Supplements that list substances such as PABA (para-aminobenzoic acid) and ubiquinone (coenzyme Q_{10}) are trading on good press from research that shows them to be essential for growth in bacteria or other life forms, rather than substantial evidence from studies in people.

Beware of potentially dangerous interactions. Pay attention to warnings on the label, and tell your doctor and pharmacist what supplements you take (see "Medications and micronutrients," page 45).

Report any serious ill effects. Let your doctor know about any side effects that you attribute to a supplement. He or she may pass along the information to FDA MedWatch, if appropriate. Or you can contact MedWatch directly at 800-FDA-1088 or through the website at www.fda.gov/medwatch/report/consumer/consumer.htm. Also inform the manufacturer or distributor and the store where you purchased it.

Resources

Organizations

Academy of Nutrition and Dietetics
(formerly the American Dietetic Association)
120 S. Riverside Plaza, Suite 2000
Chicago, IL 60606
800-877-1600 (toll-free)
www.eatright.org

This national organization of food and nutrition professionals has an extensive website offering consumers information on health, food, and fitness. You'll find a treasure trove of consumer tips, nutrition fact sheets, and healthy recipes, along with nutrition information about the Dietary Guidelines for Americans and how to meet recommendations for vitamin and mineral intake through healthy food choices.

American Cancer Society (ACS)
250 Williams St. NW
Atlanta, GA 30303
800-227-2345 (toll-free)
www.cancer.org

This website of this pre-eminent cancer organization offers a wealth of information on cancer risk, treatment, and research. Go to the "Stay Healthy" tab, then click on "Eat Healthy and Get Active" to find the ACS recommendations for healthy eating and exercise that can help reduce cancer risk.

American Heart Association (AHA)
7272 Greenville Ave.
Dallas, TX 75231
800-242-8721 (toll-free)
www.heart.org/en/healthy-living

Under the AHA's "Healthy for Good" listing, you'll find a wealth of articles and quizzes on healthy eating at home and in restaurants along with simple heart-healthy cooking techniques and recipes.

Center for Food Safety & Applied Nutrition
Food and Drug Administration (FDA)
5100 Campus Drive
College Park, MD 20740
888-723-3366 (toll-free)
www.fda.gov/AboutFDA/CentersOffices/OfficeofFoods/CFSAN

The consumer advice section of the FDA's website is your go-to site for information on dietary supplements and the Dietary Supplement Health and Education Act of 1994. The website and toll-free hotline offer information, including warnings and recalls, about dietary supplements and other products. You can also report problems with foods and supplements via the website.

ConsumerLab.com
333 Mamaroneck Ave.
White Plains, NY 10605
914-722-9149
www.consumerlab.com

If you're looking for comprehensive reviews of herbs and supplements, this subscription service offers sound advice with rankings and grades—sort of like a *Consumer Reports* for supplements. It provides in-depth information about products, recalls, and warnings, and summaries listed by medical condition.

National Academies of Sciences, Engineering, and Medicine
500 Fifth St. NW
Washington, DC 20001
202-334-2000
www.nas.edu/nrc

This is the umbrella group that includes the Health and Medicine Division (formerly called the Institute of Medicine or IOM), which oversees guidelines for nutrient intakes. You can purchase reports on a variety of nutrition topics or read them for free online.

National Center for Complementary and Integrative Health
9000 Rockville Pike
Bethesda, MD 20892
888-644-6226 (toll-free)
www.nccih.nih.gov

Part of the National Institutes of Health, this government agency is a great resource if you're looking for publications and research on dietary supplements, including herbal medicines. You may speak to an information specialist from 8:30 a.m. to 5 p.m. ET, Monday through Friday, or request information by filling out the online comment form or sending an email to nccih-info@mail.nih.gov.

U.S. Department of Health and Human Services
Office of Disease Prevention and Health Promotion
1101 Wootton Parkway, Suite LL100
Rockville, MD 20852
https://health.gov

This consumer website from the U.S. Department of Health and Human Services offers information on various aspects of a healthy lifestyle. Go to "Food and Nutrition," then "2015–2020 Dietary Guidelines," for the most recent version of the Dietary Guidelines.

Publications

The following publications provide additional information about topics in this report. To order, call 877-649-9457 (toll-free), or go online to www.health.harvard.edu.

The Benefits of Probiotics
W. Allan Walker, M.D., Medical Editor
(Harvard Medical School, 2018)

This digital publication reviews the scientific evidence for probiotics. It catalogs the different strains and species and what they're helpful for, and explains ways to get more probiotics in your diet.

The Harvard Medical School 6-Week Plan for Healthy Eating
Teresa Fung, Sc.D., R.D., L.D.N., and Kathy McManus, M.S., R.D., L.D.N., Nutrition Editors
(Harvard Medical School, 2015)

This Special Health Report from Harvard Medical School shows you how to implement doable, healthy changes in your diet one week at a time. It also contains 17 recipes for success.

Healthy Eating: A Guide to the New Nutrition
Teresa Fung, Sc.D., R.D., L.D.N., Faculty Editor, and Sharon Palmer, R.D.N., Nutrition Editor
(Harvard Medical School, 2016)

This Special Health Report helps you choose the right foods for maximum health. It includes well-researched, specific recommendations on meal planning, beverages, and snacks, plus 16 recipes.